Yoga for Skilful Living

with Yoga Satsanga Ashram, Wales

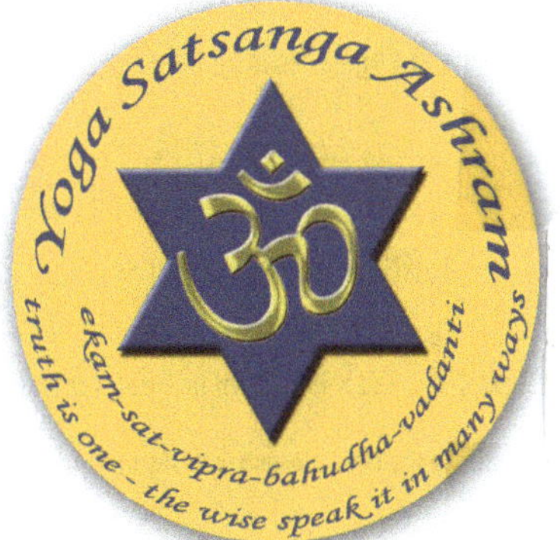

Yogacharyia Jnandev

www.yogasatsang.org

Yoga for Skilful Living

Contents:

1.1 Ethical approaches in Yoga as holistic therapy

Yogic lifestyle, health and well-being is based on strong foundations of ethical values in its first two stages, out of eight, in the Ashtanga Yoga of Patanjali. Yamas and Niyamas are codes of conduct for self-discipline to overcome our animal behaviors. Health and wellbeing, as well as spiritual evolution/freedom is only achieved through discipline. We all have to follow discipline in our actions, speech, thoughts, emotions and spiritual activities.

The five yamas, or self-regulating behaviours involving our interactions within ourselves and with other people, as well as our material world or mother nature include:

- Ahimsa: non-violence, kindness, love compassion and for ourselves and others
- Satya: truthfulness, honesty, being realistic, letting go of our judgemental conditioning
- Asteya: non-stealing and not allowing others to steal from us on physical, mental, emotional as well as material levels
- Brahmacharya: Following the laws of nature (often interpreted as celibacy), having responsibility, respect and gratitude in each and every action
- Aparigraha: non-possessiveness, non-greed, not exploiting and not letting others exploit our body, mind and emotions, as well as our mother nature or resources

The five niyamas, personal practices that relate to our inner and external world, include:

- Saucha: purity, maintaining cleanliness of body, mind, emotions and our physical surroundings
- Santosha: contentment, self-satisfaction, 'doing our best and leaving the rest', putting all our energy in our actions and not the outcomes or fruits
- Tapas: self-discipline, regularity, rhythm and repetition of practice with sincerity, faith and discipline
- Svadhyaya: self-study, inner exploration, knowing our self as we are, our body, mind and emotions, acknowledging our limits and strengths and using strengths to improve our weakness
- Ishvara Pranidhana: surrender (to God), seeing the higher reality beyond our limited perception

All these morals one needs to practice towards oneself, others and our mother nature in every situation, and every aspect beyond limitations and discrimination. Learning to be kind to ourselves and honest is not easy to practice in the beginning. Your kindness and honesty towards yourself can be accepting your limitations, resources and time limits.

1.2 Contraindication's to Yoga

Yoga as practice, tools, path, and goal is holistic in all aspects and it aims to bring us back to our true nature. Practices are designed to balance and re-establish our harmony of body, mind and soul. Our hormones can be balanced; and our autonomic nervous system will be also balanced. It enables us to become more and more conscious and responsible for our action and energy.

In the true sense yogic practices are meant to prevent the miseries yet to come. As long as you are fully aware and responsible to your practice there are not really any contraindication to Yoga. Lets say if you are suffering with back pain, all the forward stretching, twisting and back bending postures can help to improve your back bone and re-establish spinal health, as long as you are not over stretching. In hatha-Yoga every posture is described as beginner, intermediate, and advanced. If some one is very flexible and strong, holding him/her in beginner postures wouldn't give much benefit, but on the other side, if some one is struggling with the beginner postures and pushing to try the advanced it wouldn't be benefiting either as they would be prone to over stretch and hurt themselves. It's all about being kind and working with our own body, mind and soul. Through your own body awareness that Yoga develops you will also be able to know when you simply need rest from physical practices altogether if for example you have sustained certain injuries, sickness etc. Yoga within itself has hundreds of tools for practice and at certain points in your life you should only practice more meditative, contemplative or less physical aspects.

If some one is too intellectual, mentally active or imaginative, they should choose to practice hatha-Yoga, karma Yoga or plenty of physical work to keep their mind busy and to fulfill their senses in nature to be calm and still and generally vice-versa. We often find those postures we do not like to practice are the ones we need the most!

1.3 How to prepare for Yoga

If you are able to create a quiet space somewhere in your own home this is ideal, keeping this place just for your own practice in a clean, ventilated room. Make sure you have everything you need so you don't need to disturb your practice once you start, ie water, blanket, loose comfortable clothes, hair tied back and make sure your space is safe, clear of clutter and things on the floor that could get in your way.

It's always good to start with a few minutes quiet sitting, to try to watch the current condition of your ever changing mind, to try to still yourself and prepare your mind to focus single-pointedly on your yogic practice. Try to feel inside where your body needs some attention and structure your practice around these points if you can. Most importantly be sure to enjoy your practice and being at one with your own body, bringing union (Yoga) between body and mind.

2.1 A brief history of Yoga

Yoga originates from India with its earliest mention in Hindu scriptures around 5000 years ago such as the Vedas and later on the chapter of the Bhagavadgeeta that is within the great epic called the Mahabharata. In these ancient scriptures Yoga is described between Arjuna and Krishna as a way of harnessing the mind, doing ones duty in life always for the greater good and gaining union with the divine or God. Yoga's roots are very much within a Hindu lifestyle. Yoga developed to its highest extent in Indian subcontinent and in later times was also considered as part of Buddhism and Jainism as they both grew out of Hinduism and its practices.

Until the 18th and 19th century Yoga was considered a spiritual practice or path for enlightenment or liberation. In 19th century Yoga spread worldwide and one or other parts of yogic life style were practiced for various reasons, like hatha-Yoga or physical postures for health and vitality, pranayama for mental and emotional cleansing and harmony, sound work for healing, Yoga postures, kriyas and pranayama for therapeutic purposes as well as in holistic approach for self-development and holistic well-being. Many Yoga schools, teachers and institutions grew worldwide and manipulated Yoga practices in healthy or unhealthy ways to label their own or self-styled so-called modern Yoga styles.

Yoga in itself is holistic and every practice and tool is complete in itself to lead some one to holistic health and well being, so every one is benefited, which ever forms they are practicing. If someone practices relaxation /shavasana every day, its going to lead to mental and emotional balance and harmony. Hormones and the autonomic nervous system will be balanced which can result in healthy psycho-physiological functioning of body systems. So if someone is suffering with hypertension yogic relaxation will help to bring it down to normal and if one is suffering with hypotension it will bring it up to normal too.

2.2. How Yoga works

How does 'stress' work on our body?

As soon as a human being faces a stressful situation, the cerebral cortex receives this message through the sense organs and sends the impulse to the hypothalamus, which in turn passes to the medulla of the adrenal gland. The two hormones, namely adrenaline and non-adrenaline are released by the adrenal gland, in the blood stream. These hormones stimulate the individual to release glucose, the sources of energy. They constrict capillaries in the skin so that it looks pale and the blood contained in them is diverted to the muscles and internal organs and the stomach stops digesting food that is not immediately necessary. The heart rate increases. The arteries constrict and as a result the blood pressure rises. All these changes equip the body for **fight- flight response.** This flight – flight response is deeply embedded in our genetic history, hence in Yoga there are many animal postures to 'take us back' to the animal state and help release much of this animal nature conditioning.

Physiology of stress

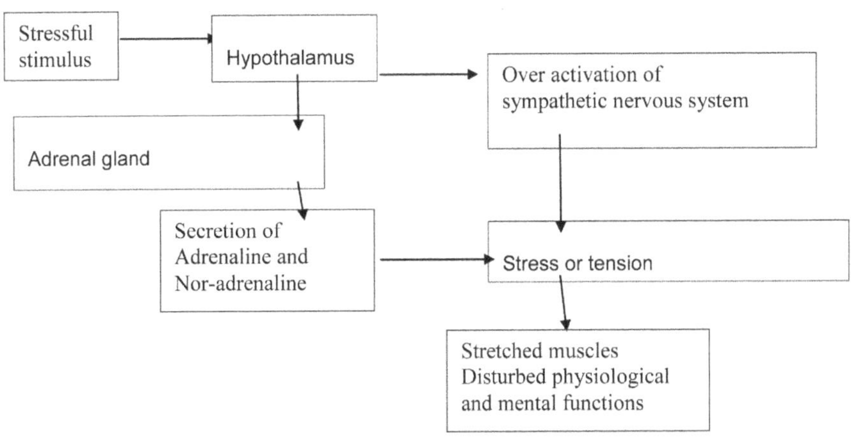

Yoga helps relaxation- In Yoga we retrain our brain to send a message to every part of the body to relax muscles, as opposed to experiencing stress. It also goes to the adrenal glands which balances the hormones. Your energy starts flowing inwardly and brings lightness, and rejuvenation. Here the sadhaka starts unfolding and unwinding all the mental and emotional stress, which you can experience after every session of your own practice.

We practice hatha-Yoga to achieve flexibility, strength and stability. We learn to let go and release all the accumulated stress, tension or burden from joints, muscles and body cells. Our prana or life force goes where ever our mind goes. Keeping your mind engaged in your own body brings your prana and life force back into your body and to work on physical, mental, emotional and spiritual level's of cleansing, healing and rejuvenating.

3.1 Benefits of Yoga

Modern aspect-   Actually Yoga is to find out ways to relax and release stress, toxins, anxieties, worries and fears that we are holding in our body and mind. We do all the movements, stretches, twists and breathing work to remove the stiffness and toxins from our joints and muscles. So our aim is to relax rather than stretch. We are doing stretches or movements of many of the muscles and joints where all the toxins are accumulated, like dust may accumulate in the corners of your house. So our stretches are to pull those muscles to their maximum length and then the movements allow us to breathe in and out in those parts of our body. So the first benefit is to help the practitioner to be free of stress. Balancing hormones will help you to cope better in different stressful and emotional situations, hence less 'trauma' for the heart and breathing. These are just a few of the many benefits. We are going to talk in more detail during our practices throughout the course.

Ancient aspect- In Hindu traditions, Yoga was part of the ashram education or practice to understand life. It was one of the paths to attain liberation, enlightenment and wisdom. It is the study of Purusha/soul/spirit and all the yogic practices can lead to Samadhi/ oneness of Purusha/soul with the Parmatman/Supreme power. *Swamiji Dr Gitananda Giriji used to say "worldly people live to learn- but the Yogi learns how to live!"*

PARTICIPANT FEEDBACK - YOGA BENEFITS FROM EU FUNDED 7 WEEK COURSE 2013.

-Yoga is here to help us find out ways to relax and release stress, toxins, worries and fears that we are holding in our body and mind
-Yoga helps to balance hormones, to help less trauma for the heart and breathing.
-Sleeping a lot better
-Having time for myself
-Made me see I do not need to hold on to my illness

GERTRUDE

-When I practice Yoga regularly the benefits are far-reaching, enabling me mentally to concentrate on being in the moment and to be truly inside myself when I practice the postures.
-The 6x3x6x3 breathing exercise practiced regularly helps to slow down and empty the mind...this is a wonderful gateway to meditation and a fantastic tool for coping with constant stress for me.
-When I practice regularly I identify the importance of relaxation, especially after stretching postures, it helps to absorb the posture work.

GILLIAN

-Yoga helps to utilizes my own energy field efficiently – retain my energy / prana. Yoga helps accept personal responsibility for energy on all levels. We open ourselves to realize our skills through seeing personal skills. Don't deny our skills – by trying to be that which we are not. We learn to stretch in order to relax, knowing our limits. Mentally, we learn to manifest positivity.

I personally appreciate Yoga for reducing stress, inducing calm, balancing /

strengthening nervousness; bringing a strong personal awareness and not judging others or fearing their opinions.

Essentially we Yoga helps to bring the integrity being-ness into everything – every action and reaction / thought and feeling.

LORRAINE

Yoga helps in
- Builds confidence and self esteem
- Ability to relax and be at one with my body
- Improve posture
- Sleep improves
- Anxiety and depression decrease
- Mood improves
- Learning a new skill to help with daily life
- Motivation increase
- Self-acceptance
- Helps to make right choice and decision
- Develop support system for mind and body

ANDREW

-Gain understanding of the principles of energy, relaxation, stress management.
-Improved mood and confidence.
-I feel that Yoga has improved the restless legs I was suffering from which kept me awake at night.
-Support system for mind and body.
-Breathing practices help centering, meditation, stress relief.

JANET

Yoga gives me a greater awareness of my body and mind and helps me to not get stuck in mental noise and emotions. It makes me feel calmer and helps me to find inner peace. It helps me get rid of stress and make the right decisions.

The breathing techniques help to calm me down and deal with problems and how to react and live in the moment.

TERESA

4.0 Techniques that can be used in Yoga

4.1 Jattis- warm ups

These are unstructured loosening up practices and can be done when ever and where ever you need, such as rolling the head, shaking the knees, legs, circling the ankles, rolling the shoulders, shaking the arms, head and whole body etc.

4.2 Kriyas or movement work with breath and awareness

Chatuspada kriya- Come to the four-footed chatus-pada-asana, by balancing your whole body on two knees and two hands with spine, neck and head straight like most of the animals. Now start walking like the tiger being aware of movements of the knees, shoulders, abdomen, buttocks and lower back.

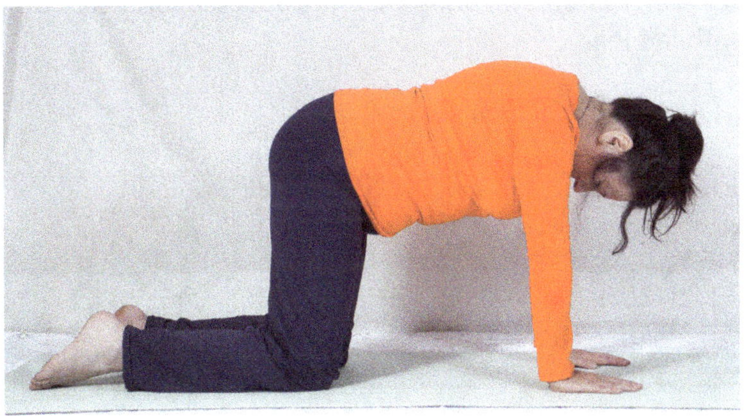

Chatus-padasana (Four footed posture)

This is very good for the digestion, knees, shoulders, kidneys, adrenal glands, uterus, and reproductive organs. This should be done for at least five minutes for desired results. This is especially recommended during pregnancy and for those who are planning for pregnancy.

Chiri-kriya 1

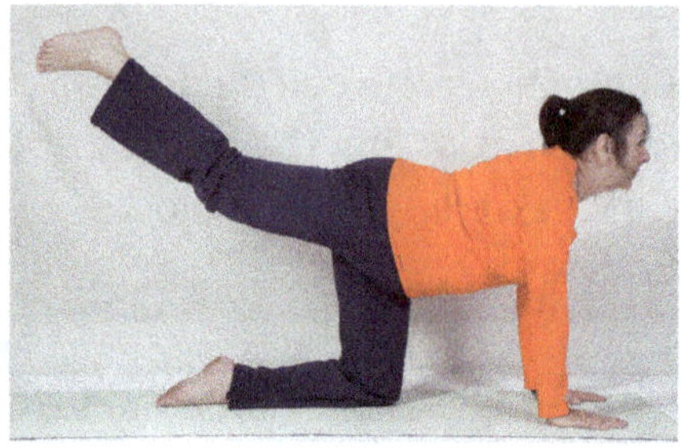 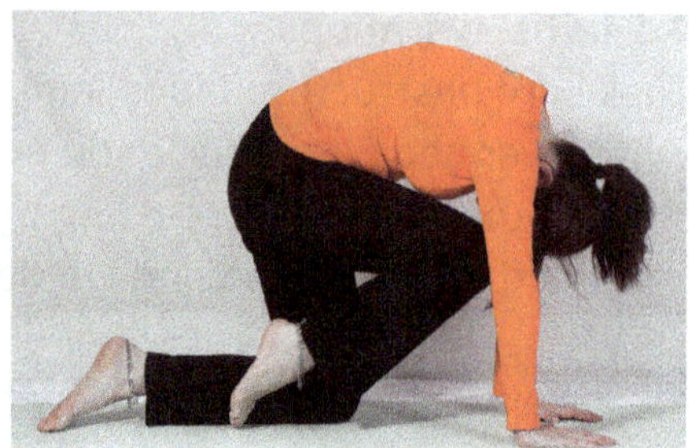

Chiri-kriya-1 and 2

Come to the chatus-pada-asana and do some deep breathing. Now with an in breath slowly stretch up your right leg behind as high as possible. With out breath, bring knee towards the forehead. Do the same with left leg.

Chiri-kriya 2 (arm variation)

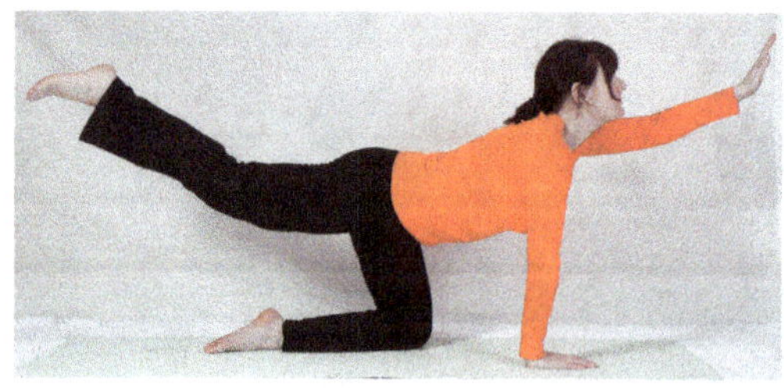 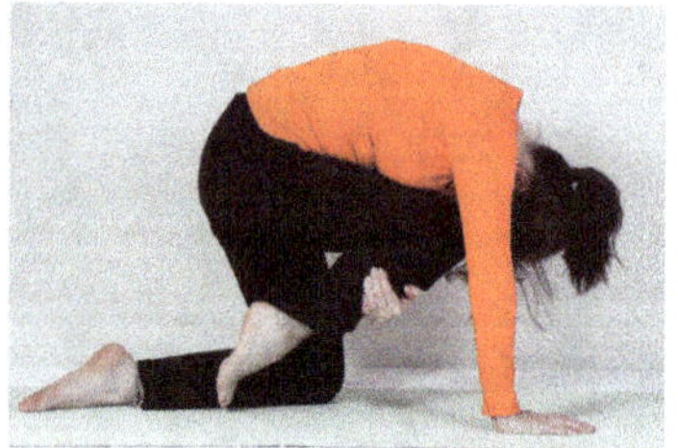

Chiri-Kriya 2

Come to the chatus-pada-asana and do some deep breathing. Now with an in breath slowly stretch up your right leg behind as high as possible, and stretch out the opposite arm. With out breath, slowly bring the leg under the body. Catch the knee, bending the knee to try and touch the knee and nose or forehad together. Stretch your back as high as possible. Return to chatus-pada-asana. Do the same with left leg.

Kokila Kriya (cookoo)

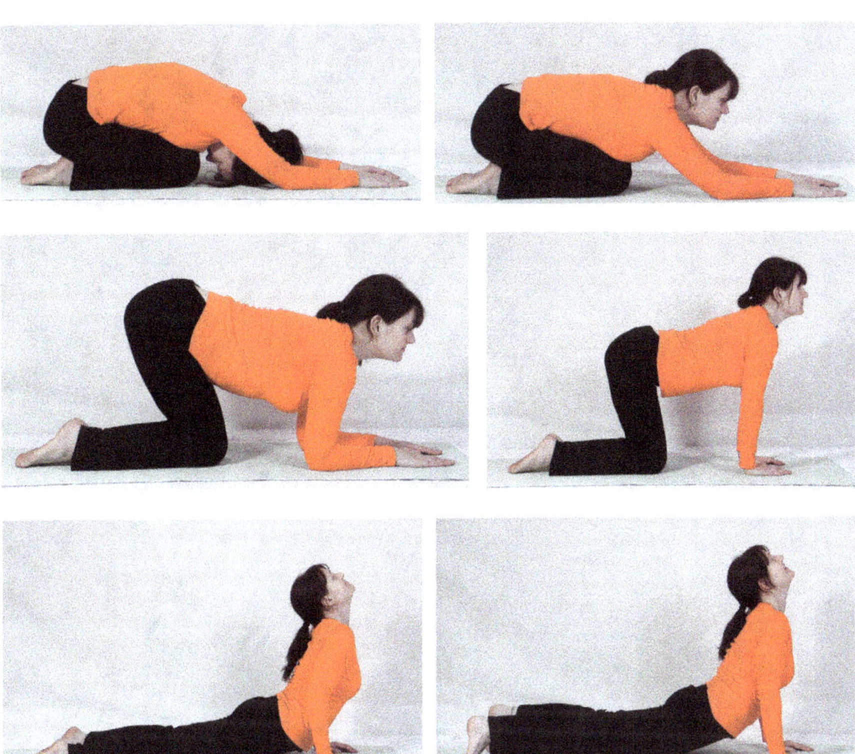

Kokila series

From Shashanka (rabbit pose) bring chin up, move forward onto elbows, then straighten arms into chatus padus (four footed) then drop the hips down into Bhujanga (cobra) and from here tuck the toes under and lift the knees (and legs off the mat) up into Kokila pose. Then come back in reverse order.

Hasta-pada Kriya

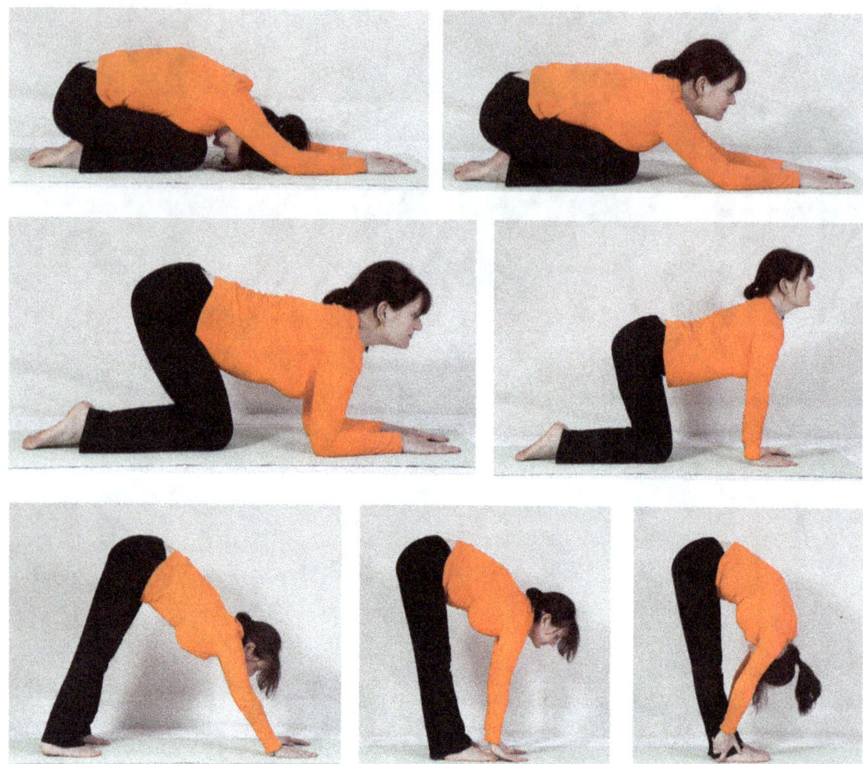

From shashanka come up to chatus padus as in previous kriya, then tuck toes under and straighten legs to push back on the heels into Meru asana (mountain pose) then start stepping forward into hasta-pada (feet to your hands) then stretch, chin up, then bring your head to your knees. Do the same in reverse order coming back to Shashanka.

Vyagraha Pranayama (Tiger breathing)

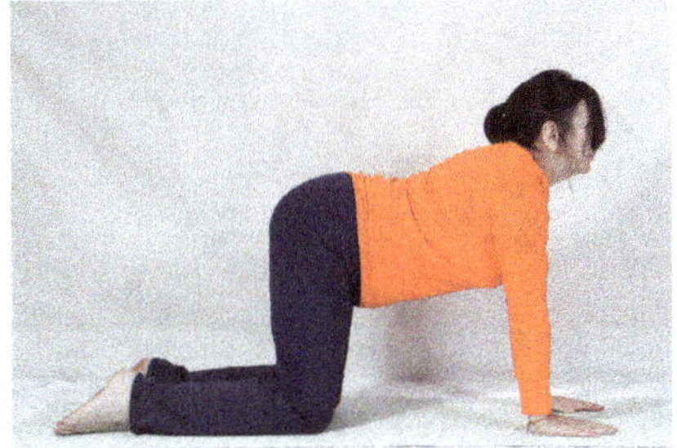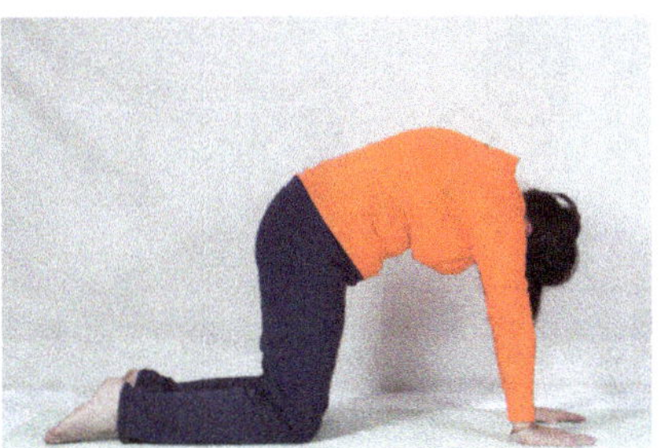

Perform the chatusa pada asana, by balancing the whole body on two hands and two knees, keeping the back straight, looking forward. While inhaling slowly raise up the head and neck, push the spine downward as much as possible. While exhaling slowly lower down the head, bend the neck down and stretch the spine upward while pulling the abdominal muscles inward.

Danda Kriya- In Sanskrita Danda means Spine or back-bone. Healthy, flexible and strong back bone signifies good health. For all breathing and meditative practices you need to have a good backbone to hold your body straight and still. Our physical, mental and emotional stress tends to accumulate in our spine and the upward flow of prana in our naris gets blocked. Danda kriya is especially good for stretching the spine, knees, neck, lungs, heart, and chest. It revitalises whole body. This is the complete balancing kriya for the prana and apana energies in the body.

Sit straight in vajrasana on your heels. The danda-kriya could be started with the shasangasana first or either with the ustra-asana. This could be performed from five rounds to nine rounds.

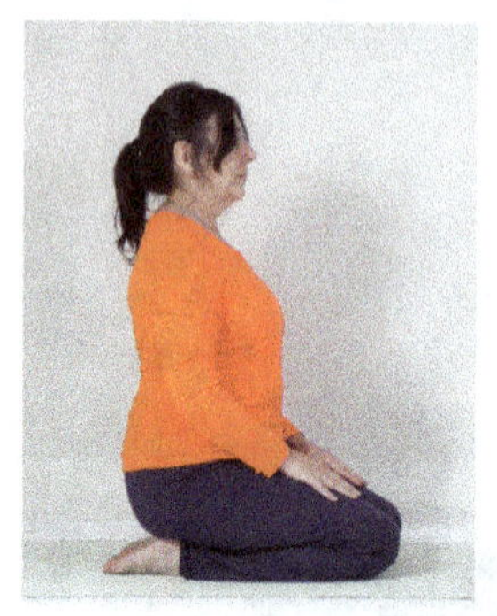 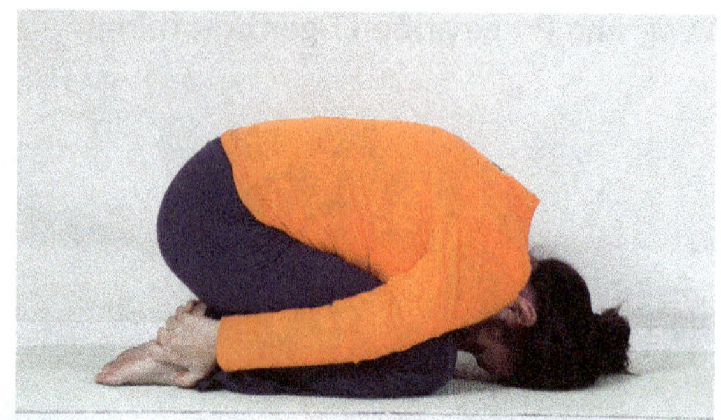

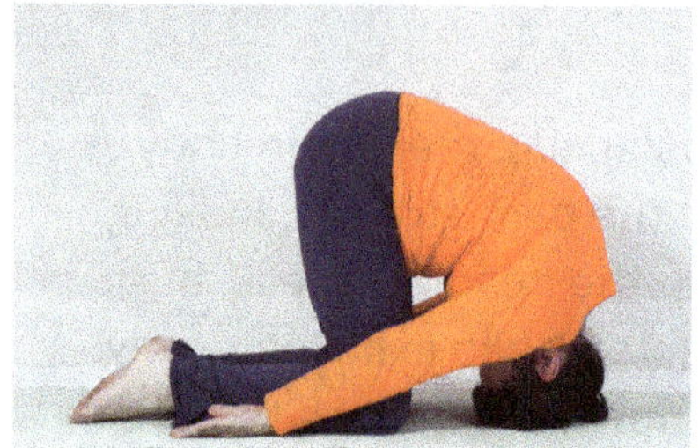 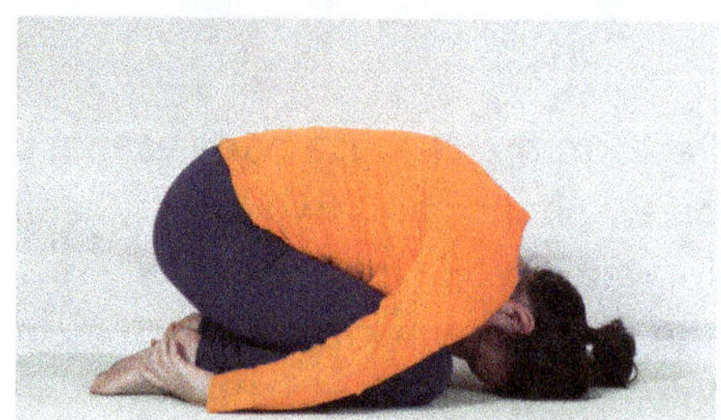

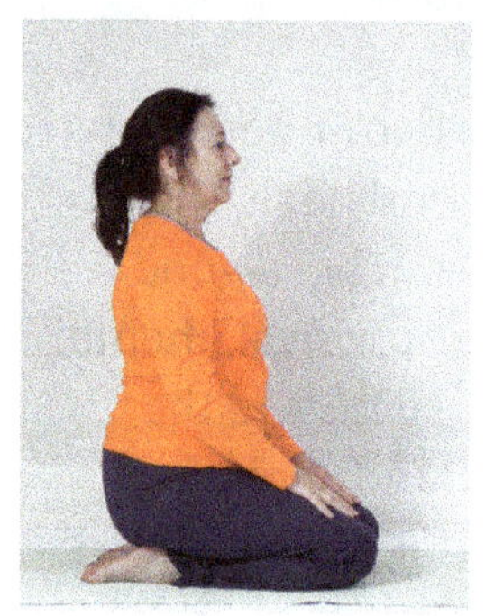 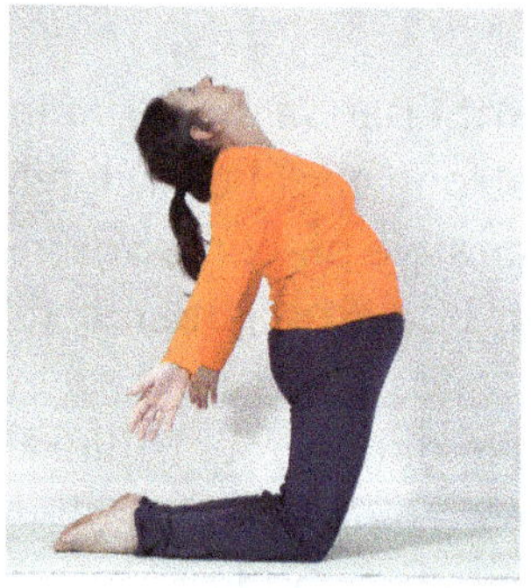 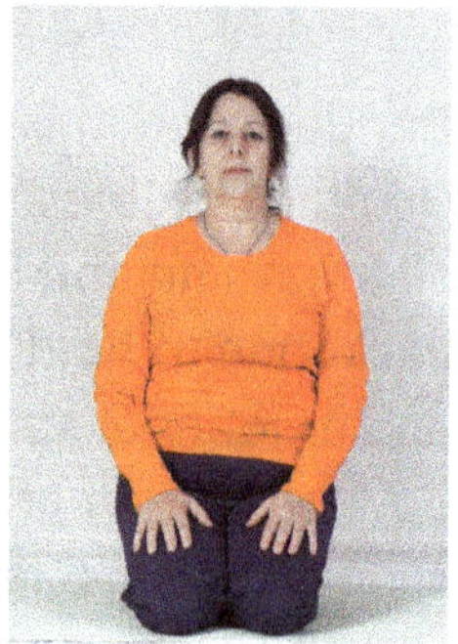

Step-I. Slowly bend forward on an in breath and place your head on the ground with nose close to the knees. Both hands should be placed on both the feet.

Step-II. Raise your buttocks high as much as you can breathing in and rolling on top of the head which will come close to your knees.

Step-III. Return back to the shasanga-asana breathing out.

Step-IV. Return to the straight vajra-asana inhaling the breath. Exhale the breath here in vajra asana.

Step-V. Slowly lift up onto your knees and bend back, inhaling the breath, opening your arms wide. This is the sapurna-ustrasana.

Step-VI. Return back to the straight vajrasana exhaling the breath. Hold vajrasana for a few normal breaths. Repeat sequence.

Pallavini Kriya These are movements for loosening up abdominal and pelvic muscles. The pelvic cavity is the most sacred part in the body as it stores the kundalini energy in the base of the spine. The abdominal cavity is the source of energy and the fire elements resides in the navel/solar plexus. In modern life these two are most misused parts in body. Stimulating and reactivating these two parts will bring a new life in your body. Many traumas and emotions tend to block energy in the pelvic and abdominal cavity and result in many digestive and pelvic disorders. In Yoga therapy Pallavini movements are best to start with. It also strengthens lower and middle back.

4.3 Asana or Posture Work for flexibility, strength and stability

Step-I. Single leg lift, Single Hand Lift

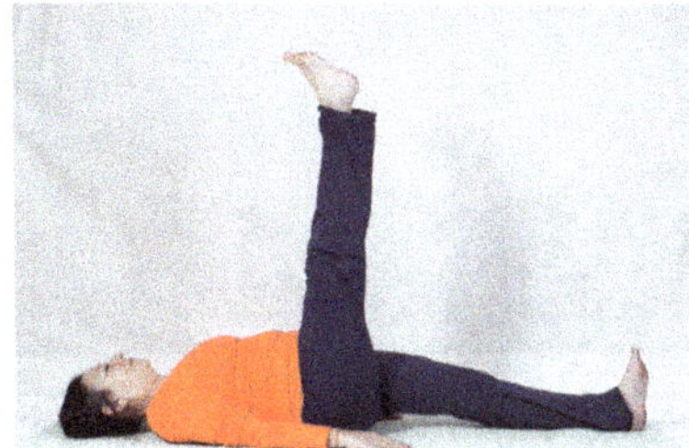 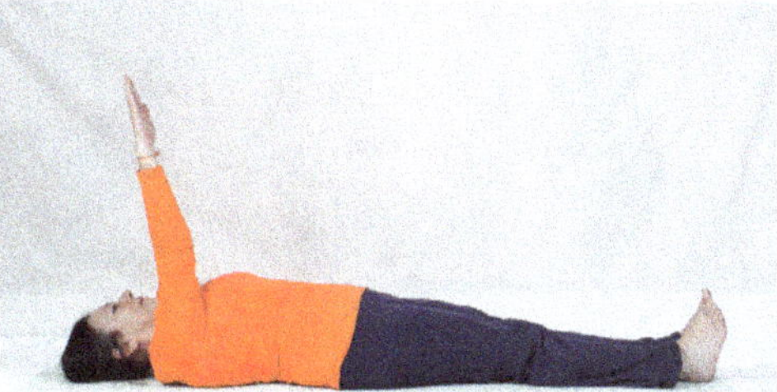

1. Lie straight in the savasana and slowly bend your right knee bringing it up to the abdomen and then straighten the leg up while breathing in. Lower down the leg after folding back during breathing out. Practice same with the left leg.

2. Now slowly lift up the right leg - keeping it straight during in breath and lower down the leg with out breath. Practice same with the left leg.

3. Now slowly lift up the right hand with keeping it straight during in breath pointing upward and lower down the hand on the out breath. Practice same with the left hand.

Step-II   One leg and one hand lift

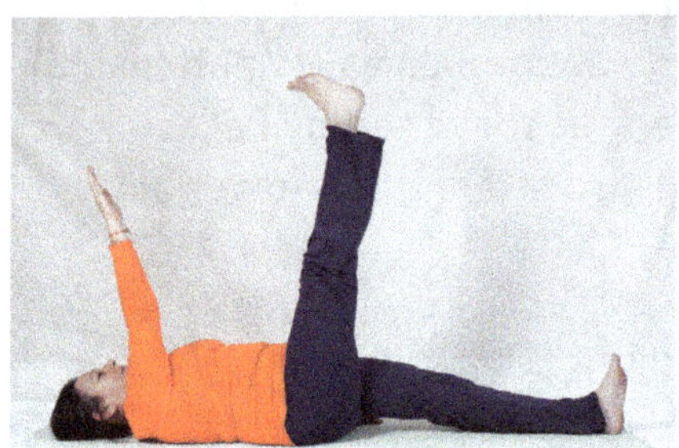
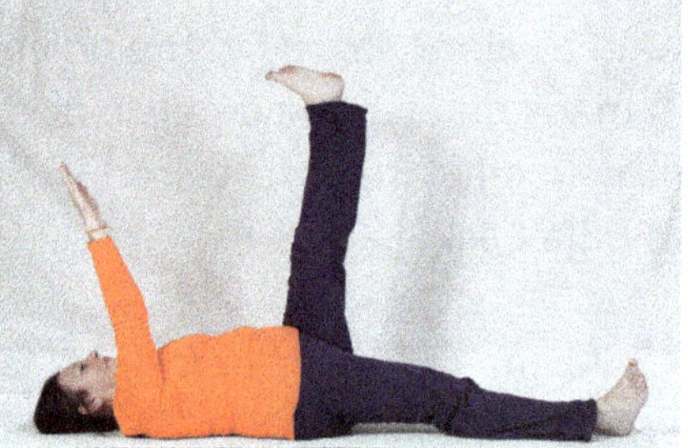

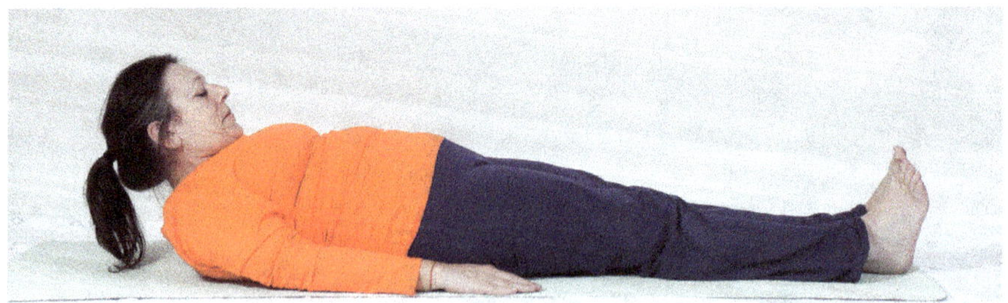

1.   Now slowly lift up the right leg and right hand simultaneously, keeping them straight during in breath and lower the leg and hand while breathing out. Practice same with the left leg and left hand.

2.   Now slowly lift up the right leg and left hand simultaneously keeping them straight during in breath and lower the leg and hand while breathing out. Practice same with the left leg and right hand.

Step-III. Head lift- Slowly raise your head up breathing in and lower your head down while breathing out.

Step-IV. Both legs lift- Now slowly lift up both legs while keeping the knees bent and then straighten up breathing in and lower the legs breathing out.

Step-V. Both hands lift- Now slowly lift up both the hands while keeping them straight during breathing in and lower the hands while breathing out.

Step-VI. Straight sit up- Slowly sit up straight in the uttana-asana without arching the back and without folding the legs breathing in. Slowly return to savasana breathing out.

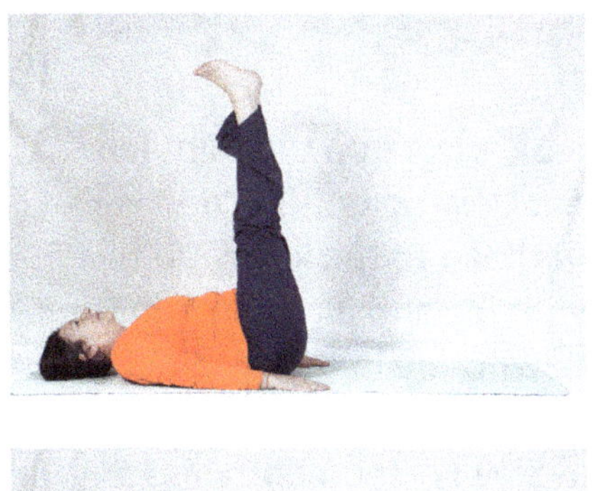
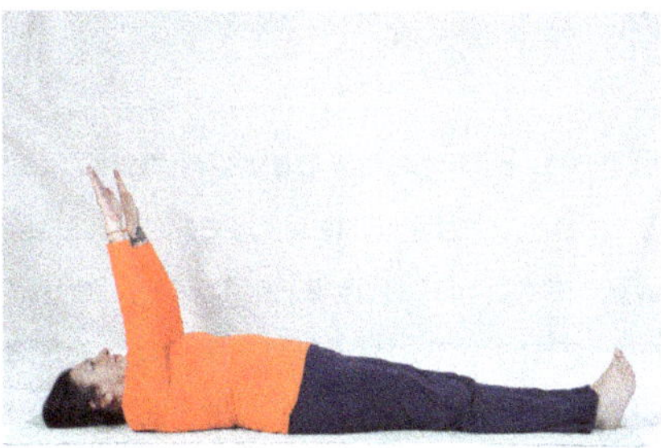
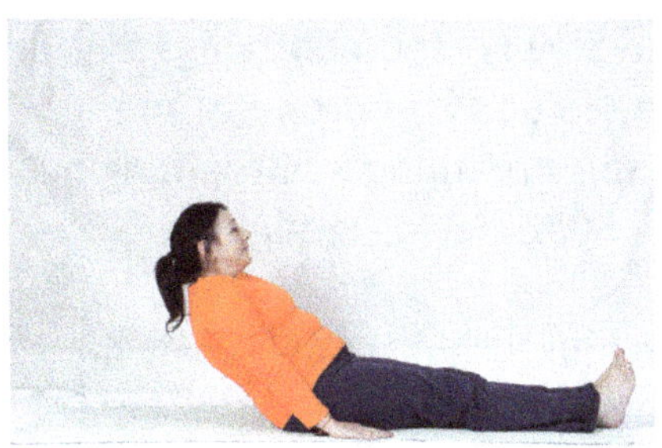
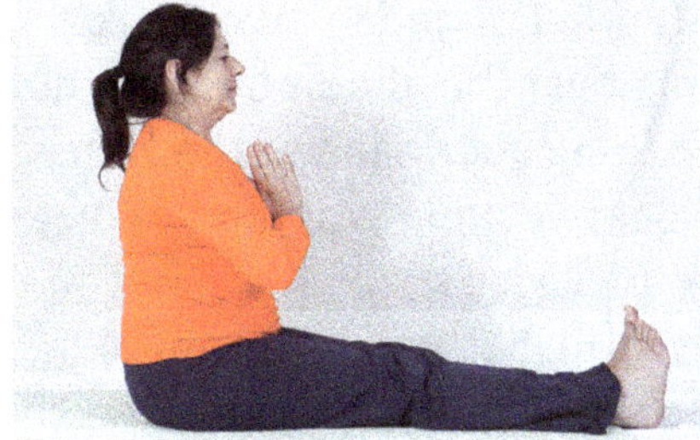

Pawanmukta kriya –Pawan is the Sanskrita term for wind also termed as 'vat' in Ayurveda. In Ayurveda and Yoga many diseases and health problems are associated with wind/pawan/vat imbalance. Wind gets trapped in our digestive canal, muscles, and naris during digestive and metabolic functions. In sanskrita 'Mukta' means to free, or release. These are movements to release wind from digestive organs, joints and muscles. Wind can be released from the body as farting, burping and sneezing for example. Don't hold any of them if you experience them during your practice. If you feel you have a wind disorder then I would recommend you do these movements, privately, regularly for few weeks without holding any wind in. You can do 3 to 6 movements with each leg.

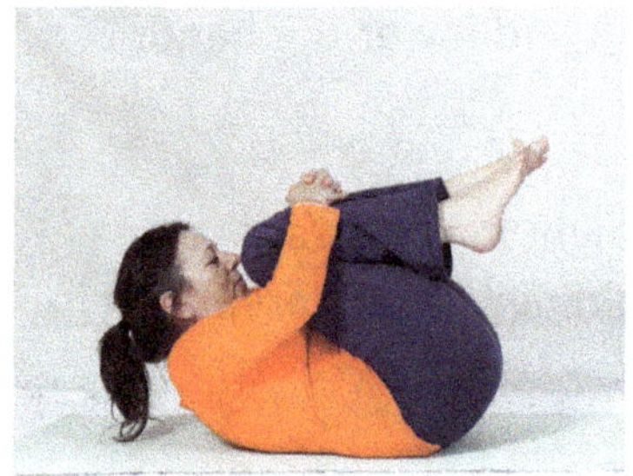 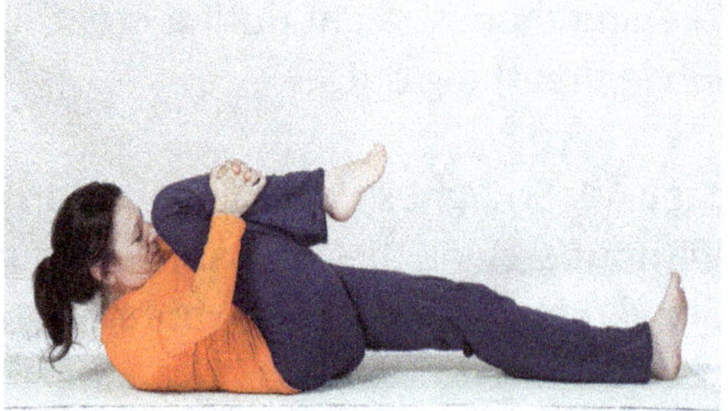

Step-I. Eka pada pawanmukta kriya- Slowly lift up the right leg and bend the knee over the abdomen. Now hold the folded leg with both hands and try to touch your head to the knee. Do this breathing in. Breathing out release your leg and place it on ground after laying straight. Repeat the same with the left leg.

Step-II. Dvi pada pawanmukta kriya- Slowly lift up both legs and fold over the abdomen. Now hold the folded legs properly and try to bring your head to the knees. Do this breathing in. Breathing out release your legs and place on ground after laying straight.

Step-III. Eka pada pawanmukta kriya mukha bhastrika- Slowly lift up the right leg and bend the knee over the abdomen. Now hold the folded leg with both hands and try to touch your head to the knee. Do this breathing in. Now vigorously kick your leg straight and open your arms wide making the loud hissing sound/ mukha bhastrika. Repeat the same with the left leg.

Step-IV. Dvi pada pawanmukta kriya with mukha bhastrika- Slowly lift up both legs and fold over the abdomen as before. Now hold the folded legs with both hands and try to touch your head to the knee. Do this breathing in. Now vigorously kick your leg straight and open you arms widely with shoulders while making the loud hissing sound/ mukha bhastrika.

4.4 Suriya Namaskars for strength and vitality

Aruna surya namaskar

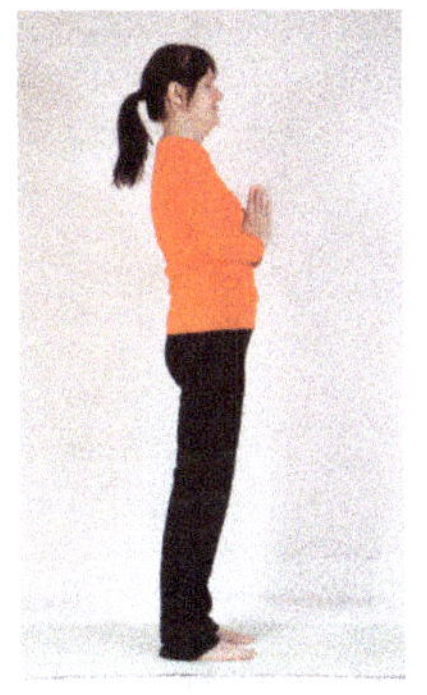
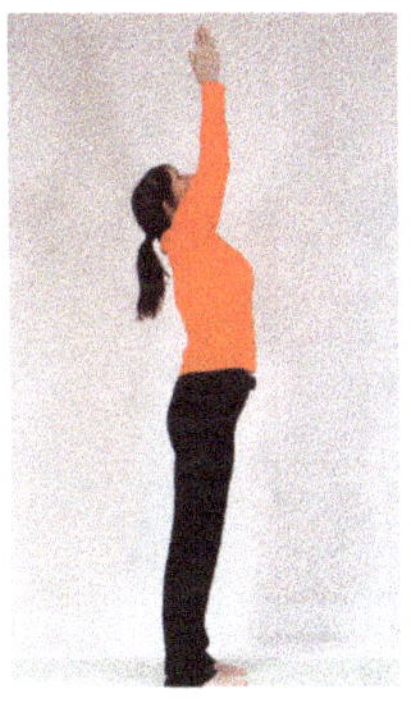
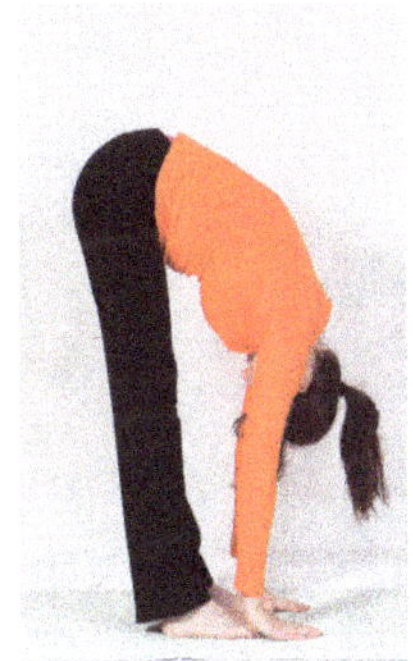
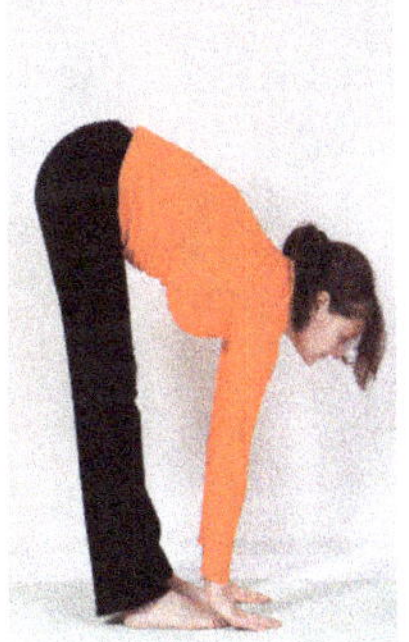
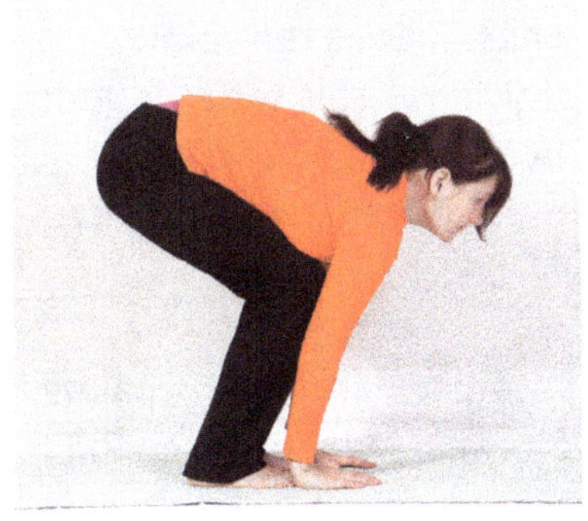
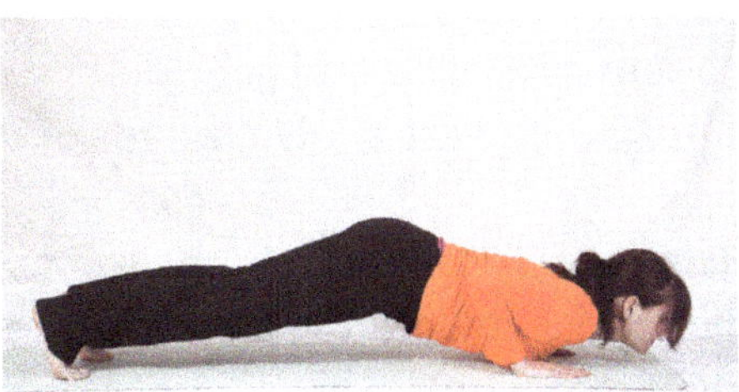

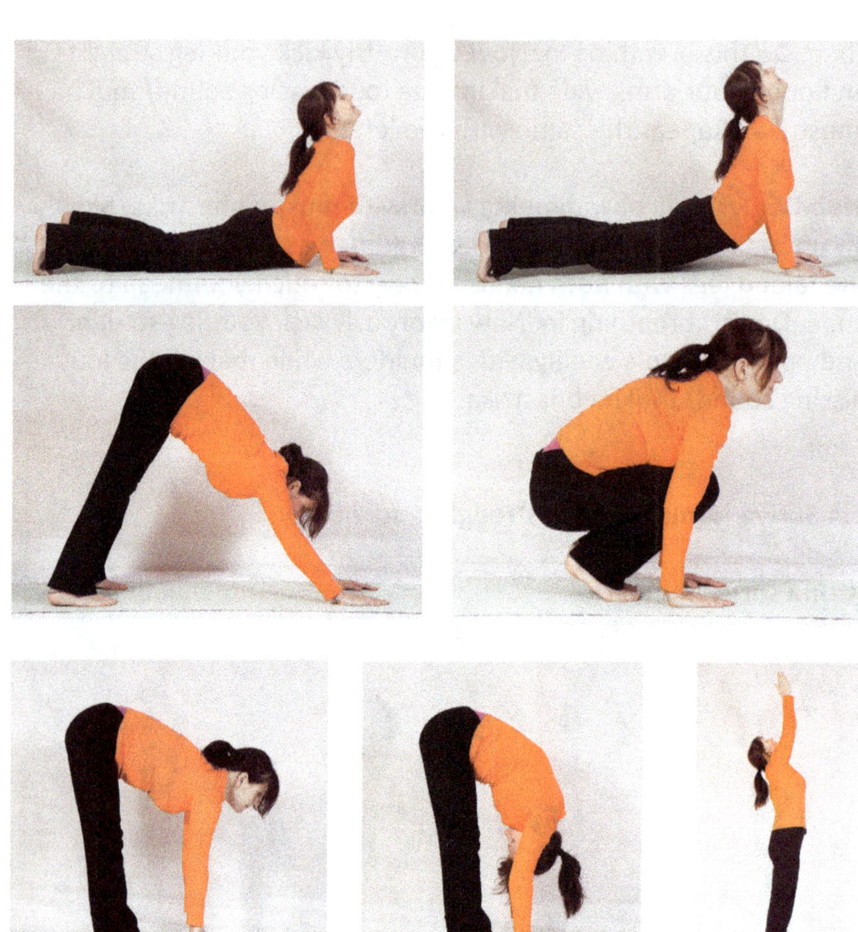

Aruna is one of the names of the sun, which means red colour. This surya namaskar has ten different positions. This series is good to gain flexibility and align the body structure. Those who wish to reduce weight and get rid of problems associated with obesity must do at least twelve rounds of it daily.

To start stand straight in the samasthiti asana while keeping palms facing out toward the sun (imagine if you can't see it but face the right direction).

Step-1. Slowly raise up both your hands in the anjali mudra while inhaling. Stretch whole body and look up to the sky.

Step-II. Open your palms to face the sun and slowly bend in front, place the palms on the ground near the feet. Touch the head to the knee while exhaling the breath. Keep your legs straight. This is hasta-pada-asana.

Step-III. Stretch your neck in front and look in front. Your spine, neck and head should become aligned in a straight position while breathing in.

Step-IV. Jump back and balance the whole of your body weight on the both hands and feet. Other parts of body should not touch the ground. Perform this while exhaling.

Step-V. Slowly raise up your head, stretch the chest upside while breathing in. Try to look the sky and keep the toes in. This is the kokila-asana.

Step-VI. Now come to meru-asana while inhaling. Balance your whole body on both hands and feet, while raising the buttocks as high as possible. Your legs and spine should be straight. Now perform a few rounds of the nasarga-mukha-bhastrika. Inhale from the nose and exhale from the mouth, with hissing sound, and exerting the diaphragm forcefully.

Step-VII. Jump forward and bring hands and feet together. Look forward while stretching the neck and spine forward then come back to the position while inhaling.

Step-VIII. Slowly bend down your head and touch the head with the knees while exhaling your breath. Your legs should be straight. This is hasta-pada-asana.

Step-IX. Slowly move up to position one, anjali mudra while inhaling and stretching the whole body.

Step-X. Slowly lower your hands and come back to the Sama-sthiti-asana, while exhaling the breath. Your palms should be facing the sun to absorb the prana and energy from the sun light.

4.5 Pranayama for cleansing of body, mind and soul

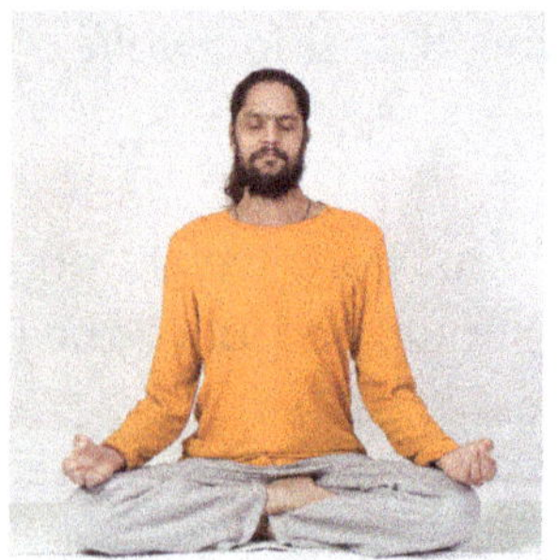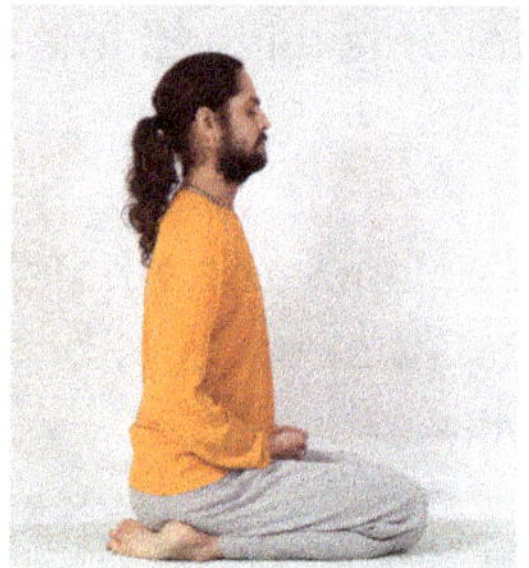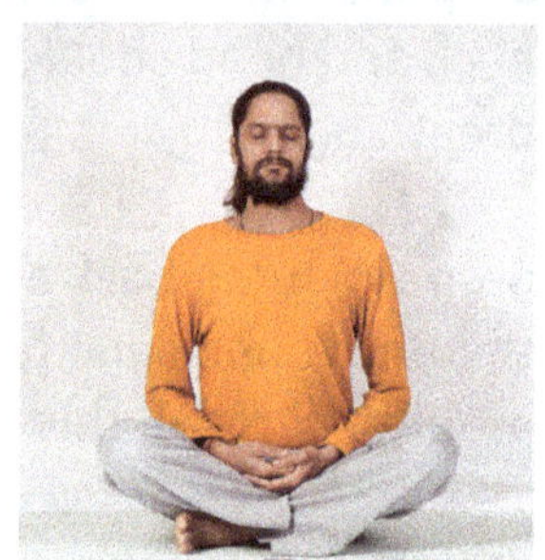

Savitri pranayama

Savitri means rhythm or harmony, thus savitri pranayama is rhythmical breathing. It brings oneness and harmony between the entire system of your body, mind, emotions and spirit. Many other terms are used in Sanskrit for this pranayama - Tulaa, mayadeyaha, shesha-avashesha, and all in some way represents the harmony. This pranayama is practiced in various timings and counts.

Here you are going to learn the classical 2x1 rhythm. The breath has four parts- inhaling, breath in known as Puraka; hold in known as kumbhaka; breath out, exhaling known as rechaka; and hold out known as the shunyaka.

Here two is for inhaling and exhaling and one is for held in and out. Simply you have to inhale and exhale in equal timings while holding in and out for half of that count. This count is known as the Tala.

If you are practicing a four Tala, it becomes 8x4x8x4, this means inhale and exhale in eight counts and hold in and out for four counts. All the talas have their own effects, like 3 tala balances the emotions, four tala strengthens and stabilizes the body, five tala increases the metabolism. The six tala increases the oxygen supply to brain, seven tala promotes serenity and peace, and eight tala is for rejuvenation. More then eight tala represents the senior or the higher practices of the pranayama.

You can practice any of the comfortable rhythm and gradually increase the talas. Twenty minutes of savitri pranayama is equal to the rest of eight hours sleep. This could be practiced in any of the classical sitting posture, like sukhasana, vajrasana, padamasana, siddhasana, or may be even in resting asanas like savasana, makarasana, etc.

Timings	Effect	Results
2x1x2x1	Increased respiratory rate Elevated blood pressure and increased heart muscle tone	No lasting effect is achieved by rapid breathing of this type. Temporary relief only of the heart muscle stress and pain.
4x2x4x2	A good rhythm for a child wishing a beneficial Pranayama, a convalescent from sickness or surgery or a heart patient wanting to correct the damage done to the heart by faulty breathing. Excellent for an asthmatic. Promotes growth by glandular stimulations.	This rhythm is of too short a duration to be beneficial over a long period of time and anyone undertaking it should try to extend the rhythm to a longer count, especially an 8x4x8x4 rhythm.
6x3x6x3	Beneficial for a narrow-chested woman or an undeveloped teenager, or an adult suffering from emotional swings, as in manic depression.	One of the best means of infusing prana into the emotional body and getting control of radical emotional swings.
8x4x8x4	This rhythm is in harmony with the cellular vibration of the blood, muscles and skeletal structure. It is the best rhythm to strengthen and rejuvenate the body.	Excellent physical health is afforded and proper electrolytic balance of the cells maintained, promoting optimum health. A good rhythm for body quietness and body meditation.
10x5x10x5	Metabolism is increased, speeding up the rate at which the body organs work. Extremely beneficial for any one with sluggish circulation and enervated nervous system.	Anyone who is constantly late and cannot get on time by other disciplines will find this routine effective. Overcomes laziness and procrastination.

12x6x12x6	The mind is awakened by a pranic flow and alertness and clearness of the senses is noted. Good for impaired sight, hearing, etc.	The student wishing to develop a good retentive memory and clearness of thought should perfect this.
14x7x14x7	The mind and senses are calmed by this rhythm. An excellent rhythm for pranic meditation.	Serenity of the mind is the by product of the rhythm. In pranayama Yoga it is called santosha pranayama, the serenity breath.
16x8x16x8	This is the siddha rhythm, the Masters Breath, and is associated with rejuvenation of the body, longevity with good health, and perfection of ideals.	Every phase of Yoga is to be mastered until one becomes a siddha or a yogi. The more difficult practices are to be learned at the appropriate time. Learn the basic rhythms and then experiment.

These rythyms are outlined by Dr Swami Gitananda Giri of our Gitananda Yoga tradition.

4.6 Jnana Yoga Kriyas or relaxation techniques

Shavasana (Complete Relaxation) _ "An Approach of Stress Management"

We all are familiar with the evidence of meditation or spiritual practices of many Yogis, they meditate in the same posture for long periods for many years. The question arises about how they live without fulfilment of physical need? Why don't they need breathing? How do they stay in the same posture? How can we develop such stability? How can we overcome the problem of stress or tension? The present discussion aims to answer all these questions.

What is stress /Tension:- In our present competitive life, stress is a fact of life. We cannot avoid it. According to **Martha Davis, et. al. (1996)**, "Stress is any change that we must adapt to, ranging from the negative extreme of actual physical danger to the exhilaration of falling in love or achieving some long desired success".

According to **Hen Selye**, "the speed of deformation in the body is known as stress". According to him temperature, anger, the environment, abuse of intoxicants, pain, fear, joy, excitement, etc., all activate the stress system and produce tension.

The differences between the two sides of the brain cause a very specific state of mind, which is called tension. Tension is a state where there is disequilibrium in the development of the right and left parts of brain. Psychologists call this underdevelopment of emotions and over development of the lower mental faculty.

According to **Spencer A. Rathus** (1994), the daily routine problems faced by a person are known as the **hassles.** The tension is developed by experiences and the daily notable conditions (daily hassles) that are threatening or harmful to a persons well being". He described these hassles in eight categories, while Gaur and Saini (2001) described these daily hassles in the various six categories, which are as follows:

1. Health hassles: e.g. physical   illness, concern about medical treatment and side effects of medication.
2. House hold hassles: e.g. preparing meals, shopping, home, maintenance, etc.
3. Environmental/ Social hassles: e.g. crime, neighbourhood, deterioration, traffic noise, etc
4. Work hassles: e.g. job satisfaction; not liking one's work duties and problems with co-workers.
5. Financial Responsibility hassles: e.g. concern about owing money, such as mortgage payments and loan instalments.
6. Others: time pressure hassles, job security problems and love affair stress.

Organisational stress- Our industries\organisations are also not free from the problem of stress. Stress has taken the role of the main obstacle in the path of efficiency, productivity, and quality in an industry. Thus stress effects growth and prosperity of an individual as well as business organisation. How?

Much research has proved that even the initial symptoms of stress like lack of concentration, irritation, unhealthy interpersonal relations, propensity to make the mistakes, indecisiveness, negative irrational thinking, consuming excessive time in the completion of the same job, getting easily frustrated, etc., can reduce the efficiency of the individuals at the levels from the chief officer to the level of the sales persons.

Easily notable adverse effects of stress in the form of psychosomatic diseases, social strains and mental weakness lead to absenteeism, increased medical bills in the organisation, lack of motivation, bad team work, low morale, etc. and all these result in poor efficiency, poor quality, less out put and reduced profits.

A research study of the **Himalayan International Institute, Honesdale, Pennsylvania, USA,** found that, "a stress free, or relaxed person is a more efficient and effective person. Sprinters run faster, students get higher scores, salesmen sell better, managers manage better, workers work harder, parents respond more wisely to their children's needs, individuals enjoy better health and prosperity. Quality of life is also improved".

Most organisations are spending a large amount of the money to develop a stress free environment, but this effort is unable to solve the problem of stress. As stress belongs to each aspect of the human life, office, work, family, etc. The change of the environment is far beyond our reach.

Many organisations have already started investing in 'stress management' for 'Human Resource Development', 'better productions' and satisfaction of employees.

Thus training in stress management as a part of the Human Resource Development program are not only a choice but also a fast emerging necessity in the industries\organisations.

Some causes of tension/stress: -

*Ill health,
 *Scarcity of memory,
*Lack of harmony,
*Unlimited desires,
*Complexes,
*Egoism,
*Declining moral values,
*Lack of trust and faith,
*Mismanagement of resources and abilities,
*Development of negative emotions like fear, possessiveness, egoism, readiness,
Jealousy, etc.,
*Over expectation from others,
*Living in the past and future,
*Always trying for better performance,
*Unhealthy life style.
*Excess work,
*Mismanagement of time
*Lack of relaxation and sleep

Some problems related to stress:

Selye's researches showed that stress or tension, particularly if it is prolonged, is very harmful to the human being. The following problems may occur due to prolonged tension.

*Heart attack.
*Brain haemorrhage.
*Digestive problems.
*Asthma and other respiratory problems.
*Headache, body ache, pain in the neck and shoulders.
*Development of negative emotions.
*Lack of awareness.
*Insomnia.
*Fatigue, weakness.
*Mental and emotional imbalance.
*Poor production
*Poor quality
*Reduced profits
*Industrial strains
*Behavioural problems

Some symptoms of Stress-

        *Stretched body muscles.
        *Dry mouth, decreased secretion of saliva.
        *Increased breathing.
        *Increased heart rate.
        *Increased blood pressure.
        *Decreased memory.
        *Lack of concentration
        *Lack of interest
        *Irritability
        *Unhealthy interpersonal relations
        *Propensity to make mistakes
        *Indecisiveness
        *Negative irrational thinking
        *Consuming excessive time in the completion of the same job
        *Getting easily frustrated,
        *Over reaction
        *Nervousness
        *Anxiety and worry.

Some physiological changes: -

1. Stretched body muscles.
2. Dry mouth, decreased secretion of saliva.
3. Decreased digestive secretions.
4. Increased metabolic rate.
5. Increased breathing.
6. Increased heart rate.
7. Increased blood pressure.
8. Increased releasing of glucose in blood.
9. Decreased neuronal activities.
10. Decreased memory.

What is Shavasana?

Yoga is the restrain of bodily movements, speech and processes of mind. Meditation means the obstruction of all the three types of activities or directing them in a particular right desired direction. Meditation is grouped in to three types – bodily meditation, verbal meditation and mental meditation. The physical or bodily meditation is the shavasana. This is also known as Kaya-gupti (steadiness of body), Kaya-sanvar, Kaya-viutsarga, Kaya-viveka (Physical restrain).

Shavasana is the process of leaving the body and awaking of the conscious (psyche). Particularly shavasana means obstruction or control of the physical external movements and activities, relaxations of all the voluntary (skeletal) muscles and reduced rate of the subtle activities, like the metabolic reactions in the cells. In this condition mental tension is released.

The precondition of mental concentration is the physical stability and relaxation. For concentration and alertness, relaxation and steadiness of body is necessary. Further the relaxation of the vocal cord is practiced, which further develops the mental stability.

Spiritual aspect of shavasana

Tension is grouped into three classes- physical tension, mental tension and emotional tension. We go for a rest when we feel tiredness. We know how to provide rest to the body. Our mind also works but we don't know how to provide rest to it.

The main cause of mental tension is irrational excessive thinking. Although thinking is necessary for a human being's well being and goal achievement, irrational or non directional thinking is the major cause of the mental and emotional problems.

To provide rest to the mind, it is necessary to learn the technique to live in the present. To live in the present means- resting the mind, leaving the heaviness and refining the mental tension.

The third type of tension is emotional tension. This is most dangerous and complicated. To get the things we like or love and to leave all that we dislike or hate is the cause of emotional tension.

The cause of materialism is excessive desires, negative thinking and mental imbalanced development. As regular practice of shavasana removes the mental and emotional stress of a person, thus spiritual development is the result.

Shavasana and energy conservation

Complete relaxation is the process of physical and mental refinement. In the waking conditions our muscles consume energy for mechanical activities. During sleep, although the muscles are in the resting state, even now they consume the energy. This can be measured by using the GSR machine, which notes down the skin resistance. This is also the cause of feelings of lethargy even after a long rest.

During the practice of shavasana, muscular activities are completely obstructed. Now the flow of electromagnetic energy is completely stopped in the muscles. Thus the energy consumption is completely obstructed and energy is conserved now.

The energy need of the cells is fulfilled by the metabolic reactions in the cells. The energy is consumed in the emotional, mental and mechanical process. During shavasana all the emotional, mental and mechanical activities are minimized, the rate of metabolism is also decreased. The result is the conservation of energy.

Shavasana and sleep -

An electro-magnetic energy flows throughout all the body muscles. This energy flow is essential for making the body's muscles work. When there is a lack of energy, we feel the need of rest. During rest or sleep this energy consumption rate is reduced and we feel better. But due to mental stress we cannot take complete rest during sleep.

Electromagnetic energy or psychic energy flows throughout the body. This flow is at maximum at the time of wakeful states. The flow is decreased during sleep. The flow of electromagnetic energy is minimised during shavasana.

In shavasana all the mental and physical activities are obstructed. We relax muscles with awareness. Now the energy flows towards the nervous system, and our mind gets rest, our thoughts are also refined. Many researches have proved that one can get the rest of 4 hours deep sleep during half an hours complete relaxation with awareness.

Death-and self realisation

Shavasana is the process of experiencing death without dying. At first, all voluntary activities are restrained and the whole body is relaxed. The breathing rate is slowed down and can be reduced to 1 or 2 breaths per minute. Now there are no feelings of the breath and body.

When all the voluntary actions are relaxed, our consciousness or prana moves inward. Now all the involuntary functions are also restrained, and when the practitioner crosses the bridge of instabilities of body and mind, he perceives the psyche or conscious. The practitioner now perceives the soul itself. The major cause of pain is the Karman body (action body), which is washed out by shavasana by physical, mental and emotional purification and stability of the mind and body.

Shavasana (relaxation) and stress management

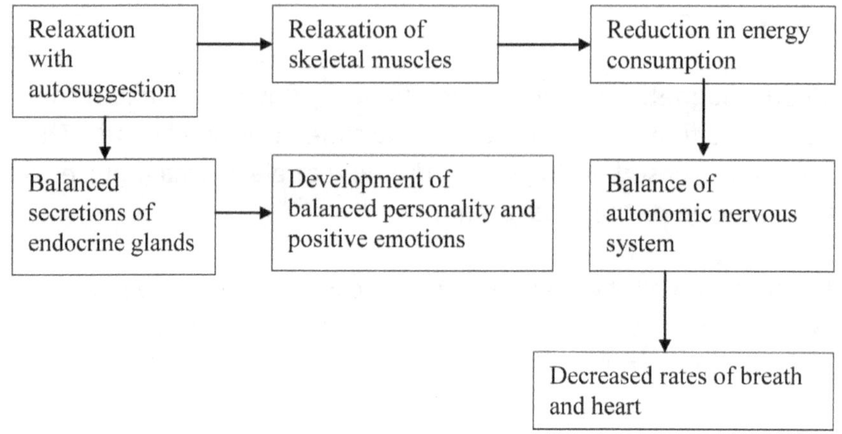

A process of relaxation

"Shavasana is the technique to release the physical, mental and emotional tension and to develop steadiness in the body".

"The basic purpose of shavasana is the awareness of the real self apart from the body, without affection, apart from the emotions and excitement".

The two necessary conditions of shavasana are (i) the total cessation of voluntary movements, that is relaxed condition of all skeletal muscles and (ii) extremely slow rate of respiration as if the system has stopped working.

The meaning of shavasana is complete relaxation with self-awareness, shavasana is an effective, harmless and easily learnable technique. Releasing the tension, one can enjoy a healthy and happy life. One, who practices relaxation for 30 to 45 minutes daily in life, would remain relaxed and unprecedented in any situation.

Gaur and Saini (2001) and **Gaur, Saini and Srivastava** (2001) have explored the effective role of preksha meditation in releasing tension and anxiety and refinement of emotions of prisoners in Central Jail, Jodhpur.

Shavasana is a better process of resting and relaxation in comparison to sleep. During muscular and physical activity, high electromagnetic current flows in the muscles, whilst during deep-sleep a weak magnetic current flows and during the relaxation (shavasana), this flow is minimised and at its perfection, it is completely stopped, hence energy is also conserved.
Shavasana and therapy

Shavasana is an effective stress management therapy for the following physical and mental problems-
- Mental weakness
- Physical weakness
- Insomnia
- Weak memory power
- Hypertension
- Heart troubles
- Respiratory problems
- Epilepsy
- Lack of concentration
- Emotional imbalance

These problems are more prominent in the case of excess stress. By regular practice of shavasana, one can release stress and attain relaxation of the mind and muscles. Energy is conserved by the practice of shavasana, thus during shavasana the energy flow is directed towards the brain and the nervous system. The nervous system is activated now and thus the neuro-endocrine control system is also activated. Immunity power is developed by regular practice of shavasana.

The secretions of the endocrine glands are also balanced by regular practice of shavasana. Excessive secretions of the adrenal hormones of the adrenal gland are responsible for the fight and flight response. This regular excessive secretion of epinephrine may lead to problems of hypertension, heart troubles, emotional imbalance, negative irrational thinking, etc. The secretions of the endocrine glands are balanced by refinement of thoughts, emotions, mind and releasing stress, thus shavasana is an effective technique for health promotion.

Physiological changes by shavasana

- Relaxed muscles.
- Decreased breathing rate
- Decreased heart rate.
- Decreased blood pressure.
- Decreased secretions of lactic acid.
- Decreased metabolic rate.
- Balanced automatic nervous system.
- Balanced hormonal functions.

Mental and emotional changes by shavasana

- Development of mental and emotional balance
- Refinement of negative thought and emotions, i.e., frustration, fear anxiety, jealousness.
- Increased memory.
- Development of happiness and joyfulness.
- Better sleep.
- Development of rational thinking.

Technique of shavasana: -

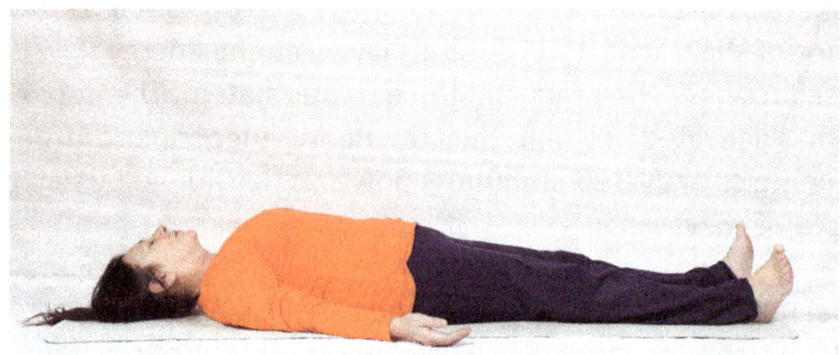

Step-1 Stretch the whole body and then relax the muscles completely; three times in standing posture and three times in the lying posture.

Step-2 Lie on the back, there should be one to two feet distance between the legs and hands should be in comfortable position apart from the body, palms in upward direction. Feel heaviness in the whole body. Feel lightness in the whole body (three times for each).

Step-3 Focus on each part of the body one by one from toe to head and suggest that each part relaxes and than feel the relaxation with awareness.

(Autosuggestion with complete awareness)

Step-4 (for spiritual development) Concentrate on the body as a whole and visualise a cool white colour around the body like the moonlight. Feel the coolness and peace of the white colour in your aura/energy layer around you.

Step-5 with two or three long deep breaths feel the activation and energy in the whole body.

5. 0 Yoga philosophy

5.1 What is Yoga?

"Yoga is the science of the sciences. Yoga is an art, a philosophy, a religion, a fad or a fanaticism." The Meaning or definition of Yoga depends on the individual person, according to their level of consciousness and evolution. Yoga can be simply described as the process to control the perception and the conceptions which develop the conscious, rational thinking and viveka (discernment).

Yoga is one of most precious jewels of the Ancient Hindu ways of attaining liberation. Even then Yoga is not concerned with religion. Yoga can help us to live with greater harmony. Today you can find people practicing Yoga everywhere. Hatha-Yoga (asanas and Pranayama) has particularly become the synonym of Yoga. So to enhance the meaning of your life, religion, faith and practice, Yoga is the tool, which is free from religion, caste or creed and available for one and all.

The term 'Yoga', which is multi-faceted and derived from the root 'yuj', generally means 'union', 'to join', 'to yoke together', or 'to unite as one'. The word Yoga comes from the most ancient language known to man; Sanskrita. In India, Sanskrit is considered to be the language of God, and is formed in a mathematical way. Yoga in India is also considered as one of the six Ancient Indian Philosophies. Primarily we should keep in mind that Yoga is the 'way of union'.

The Bhagavadgeeta uses it (i.i.48) to mean sole desire for supreme divinity (paramesvarikaparata- sridharasvamin). In i.i. 50 of the same treatise, Yoga denotes skill in work (karmasu kausalam). In IV. 1,2,3, Yoga means Karma Yoga (desire less action) and JnanaYoga (acquisition of time knowledge). In VI. 16, 17, the term Yoga means Samadhi in which the mind is united with the Atman. In VI. 23, Yoga means a state of mind, which having realized the Supreme Being, is not disturbed even by great suffering. In i.i. 48 and vi. 33, 36, Yoga means samatva or equanimity, i.e., indifference to pleasure and pain.

Yoga can be accepted as a way of life, a way of integrating your whole awareness with the true nature of the Self. Physical, mental, emotional and spiritual aspects of your life should work in integrated harmony with each other.

In arithmetic, Yoga means addition. In astronomy it means

conjunction, lucky conjunction and also conjunctions which may warn of danger, etc.

In the Upanishads, Yoga generally means union; union of Jivatman with Parmatman. Patanjali in his Yoga Sutra (i.2) defines Yoga as "Yogah-chittavrattinirodha", this means control of the whirlpools of the mind. By Yoga, Patanjali means the effort to attain union, or oneness of Self with the Supreme Self.

What is union? In the normal sense of Yoga this union means harmony of the body, mind, emotions and spirit. It is living in the present, moving and accepting all situations as they are with a positive attitude.

The Devata-smati says
"visayebhyo nivartyabhi-preterthe manasovasthapanam Yogah".
Yoga means fixing the mind on the desired object.

According to Daksha-smriti, Yoga is as follows-
      "vrittihinam manah krtva ksetrajnahparmatmani
        ekikrtya vimucyate Yoganam mukhya ucyate."
One who is aware of the soul, having turned the mind, which is rendered devoid of function, solely to the Supreme Soul, is liberated; this is called principal Yoga.

The Vishnupurana defines Yoga-
      "atman-prayatna-sapeksa visista ya manogatih,
        tasya brahamani samYoga Yoga ityabhidhiyate."
The connection of that special course of mind, which depends upon one's own effort, with Brahma is called Yoga.

5.2 Yoga as Four-fold Awareness

Our Ancient Rishis/ Sadhus/ Saints taught that oneness already exists, but that we are unaware of this state of union. So we see the duality, multiplicity everywhere. **Most of our awareness is diverted to search out the differences between one and another,**

in place of seeing unity. Our Yoga approach is to attain that Advaitaik, or state of non-duality.

Yoga teaches a four-fold awareness. **Yoga is conscious evolution.** Our evolution rests in our own hands and it must be conscious, through sensitive awareness. Thus the yamas and niyamas must be learned consciously. Initially you may start with the gross awareness of the body and later on turn to the awareness of the mind and emotions. It may become too strenuous for you to know your true self- image.

The first stage is awareness of the body and how it works, how to care for it, how to love it, how to worship it. We all want to be healthy but we are living with unawareness in regard to our health, or cannot make the necessary efforts required! Only health begets health. Try to develop the consciousness about right healthy diet, right exercise, right breathing, right rest and relaxation. This includes the complete awareness of all your physical activities going on continuously.

The second stage is awareness of the effect of the emotions upon the body. Most of us are indulged in negative destructive emotions. Try to be aware of them and their destructive effects on your body. Hate, anger, lust, greed, aversion, envy, irritation, etc are causes of all psychosomatic diseases, which result in serious illness. Destructive emotions have a powerful detrimental effect upon the body. Serenity, love, compassion, empathy, understanding, etc have a powerful positive effect on our body; Right emotions have a beneficial, healing effect upon the body. You may use many of the relaxation techniques and pratyahara kriyas to develop this awareness.

The third stage is awareness of the mind and how the mind can control the emotions and the body. Adhi-Vyadhi is the sanskirit term for all diseases, which originate in your mind and manifest in your body. It is the term for psychosomatics in modern medical science.   When the phase is accomplished, a new awareness can be sought, one in which the conscious mind is transcended by a higher aspect of the mind called Buddhi. Dharana, concentration and Dhyana, meditation are used to produce this awareness.

The fourth stage is "awareness of awareness" described as Samadhi or Cosmic Consciousness. I heartily pray to my Guru Swami Gitanada Giri Gurumaharajji to give us strength and ability to attain this stage of Samadhi.

Meenakshi Devi Bhavanani adds the fifth awareness to this four-fold awareness of Swamiji. That is the awareness of how unaware we are. To begin to walk on the path of awareness we need motivation and this can be enhanced once we come to know and recognise our unawareness.

Now you need to inculcate that awareness. Try to be aware of work, movements, walking, resting, eating, and talking. During Hatha Yoga practice be aware of your movements, stretching and relaxation, twists, body organs effected, sensations and stimulations, etc.

Don't be afraid of your ego, dullness, negative thoughts and emotions. You need to transcend them to grow on the path of evolution. Watch out if any pain is there. Watch out if there is any stress or strain. Watch out if there is any sorrow or negative emotion. You may observe your breath, heart beats, movement of the diaphragm with the breath, and try to keep the mind concentrated in the body.

Know your each thought and emotion. Whenever you have negative thoughts or emotions you may use the mental repetition of om shanti, om shanti (Om Peace). There may be arousal of some spiritual experiences during the quietness of the mind and emotions.

Try to notice your sleep. If you have a sleep disorder you may use the Yoga-nidra or relaxation exercise before going to sleep. If possible try to develop the awareness of your dreams. This will develop the insight required for higher Yoga in you.

Try to recall your good memories and develop a positive attitude regarding your self image. Always feel self-satisfied with what you have done. Feel gratitude for what you have. In Geeta Lord Krishna says that you do your duties and don't be worried for the fruits. Simply we conclude with the thought- **"do your (absolute) best and leave the rest."**

5.3 Panchavrittis for understanding states of mind and learn how to deal with our individual mental and emotional stuff

The first approach towards evolution is to understand nature and states of mind. To transcend you need to know what you want to transcend. Maharishi Patanjali describing as follows-

Yogah chitta vritti nirodhah.
Yoga is the mastery of the activities of the mind-field and stilling whirlpools of mind.
Tada drashtuh svarupe avasthanam.
Then the seer rests in its true nature.Then the seer/sadhaka/ practitioner is one with the Supreme Power/God/pure consciousness.

Yoga categorize thoughts or mental modifications in five categories. These are root cause of klishta/bad and aklishta/good in our life; pain and pleasure, suffering and joy. These are:

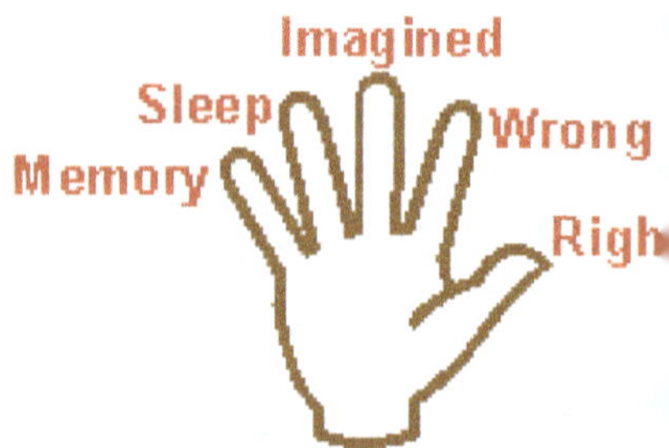

1. Pramana - real or approved cognition, right knowledge, valid proof, seeing clearly. This can be by means of direct perception, inference and from words(listening and studying scriptures). Pramana is the one to be cultivated by seeing all everything as they are, without conditions or afflictions of mind.

Keep watching your own mind whenever you can, with letting go and not holding/suppressing thoughts and emotions to attain ekagra and nirodhah states of mind. Allowing yourself to change for better and not allowing to be fixed in one or other way as things can be done differently.

2. Viparyaya - unreal cognition, indiscrimination, perverse cognition, wrong knowledge, misconception, incorrect knowing, not seeing clearly. This is similar to ignorance. Example- Seeing a snake in a rope due to lack of light. Its like we assume that no one likes me or people look down at me and judging me in negative way. Once we become negative or fixed in that kind of mental perceptions everything seems to be going against us. Try to open your heart and stop worrying about what others are thinking or talking about you, just like you every one is busy in their own mental and emotional whirlpools.

3. Vikalpa -imagination, verbal misconception or delusion, fantasy, hallucination. Vikalpah is source of ignorance /avidya. This is situation when one creates its own objects by words and imagination even though the object doesn't exist. Its like imagining what will happen if I loose my job or partner and you whole psycho-physiology has to suffer with it as if it happened in reality. Stop wasting your time into imaginative negativity and use this energy into creative things you can do.

Jnana Yoga Kriya-1 (Pramana). When you are trying to relax or meditate try not to force, imagine or create something you are intending to experience as it may result into viprayaya or vikalpa.

Allow your mind to calm down and attain stillness by watching, or observing your mental activities without being effected or judging with conditioned mind.

4. Nidra - deep sleep. Deep sleep or nidra is also stated as a negative modification of the mind. During this mental state the mind is overcome with heaviness and no other activities are present. This state is virtually a withdrawal from the external world, when one is left without any control over one`s consciousness. The dream state and the conscious state are not modifications because while dreaming, our minds are occupied with vikalpa and while awake, the mind is concerned with the categories of pramana and viparyaya. Don't let yourself to be indulged or drown into the state of not knowing what's going on in your body and mind. Be responsible, stand on your feet and don't let others walk on your shoulders.

5. Smriti- memory, remembering. This is concerned with the evocation of stored impressions, or rather the mental retention of conscious experiences. All these modifications of mind can be in any of the five states of mind. Use your memory to remember all the good and positive things in your life to build your self-confidence and positive attitude. Let your memories becomes your experiences and strengths to be able to deal better and better with every life situations.

5.4 Five modifications of Mind and Self-development

Otherwise identified with whirlpools of mind and degrees of destruction.
Depending on the degree of distraction, Yoga philosophy categorizes the mind under five stages of being:

- Kshipta or disturbed,
- Mudha or stupefied,
- Vikshipta or distorted,
- Ekagra or focused, one pointed and
- Niruddha or the absolutely balanced state of mind.

1. Kshipta/disturbed / distracted: The ksihipta state is disturbed, restless, troubled, wandering state of mind. It might be severely disturbed, moderately disturbed, or mildly disturbed. It might be worried, troubled, or chaotic. In this stage one still have some control or awareness of mind/thoughts.

2. Mudha/dull: The mudha mind is stupefied, dull, heavy, forgetful. This stage of total inertia, it is like being in crowd, noise and dark where you one is unable to sense anything. It is a dull or sleepy state, somewhat like one experiences when depressed. It is state where one doesn't want to do anything, unable to think, or move.

3. Vikshipta/distorted / damaged: The Vikshipta is distracted state of mind. This is like when you trying to sit down quietly and meditate. Every time you realise, you found your mind running here and there and drawn into chain of unbroken thoughts, and memories. This is termed as drunken monkey mind beaten by a scorpion.

4. Ekagra/single/one-pointed: The Ekagra mind is one-pointed, focused, and concentrated on the desired point. This is beginning of meditation. Here mind is undisturbed, and unaffected with external and internal stimulus. This is stage of complete physical, mental, emotional awareness.

5. Nirodhah/mastered: The Nirodhah is stage of stillness, quietness, refined and pure mind. This is stage oneness of body, mind and spirit. The word Nirodhah can be translated as controlled, regulated, or restrained, but this not state of suppression of thoughts and emotions. It is state where thoughts and emotions are not any more. Here sense organs, mind and consciousness flow inward in heart, pure bliss, joy, freedom.

What to do? We all find ourselves in one or other states mentioned above. These are natural states we all go through in various situations due to external and or internal stimulus or situations. We all are masters or hanging or clinging to one or other states of mind. too much indulgence in negativity results in depression, low mood, hormonal imbalance, lack of interest, etc. It is like when you do anything wrong or a failure in life, you keep repeating and reminding to yourself 100s of times. On other hand how many times do you repeat all the good things you have done to yourself or other people? Learn to appreciate, respect and be grateful to each and every moment of your life will help you to live more and more in higher states of mind.

5.5 Ayurvedic Diet and Health

According to the ayurveda, medicines and foods are sattvic, rajasic or tamasic or a combination of these gunas.The gunas are three fundamental attributes that represent the natural evolutionary process through which the subtle becomes gross. In turn, gross objects, by action and interaction among themselves, may again become subtle. Thus the three gunas are defined as :

Sattva : Essence (subtle)
Rajas : Activity
Tamas : Inertia (gross)

People equally can be more or less dominated by one of the three gunas and an important way to regulate these gunas in body and mind is through ayurvedic cooking :

Sattvic foods :

- Are fresh, juicy, light, unctuous, nourishing, sweet and tasty.
- Give the necessary energy to the body without taxing it.
- The foundation of higher states of consciousness.
- Examples : juicy fruits, fresh vegetables that are easily digestible, fresh milk and butter, whole soaked or also sprouted beans, grains and nuts, many herbs and spices in the right combinations with other foods,...

Rajasic foods :

- Are bitter, sour, salty, pungent, hot and dry.
- Increase the speed and excitement of the human organism.
- The foundation of motion, activity and pain.
- Examples : sattvic foods that have been fried in oil or cooked too much or eaten in excess, specific foods and spices that are strongly exciting, ...

Tamasic Foods :

- Are dry, old, decaying, distasteful and/or unpalatable.
- Consume a large amount of energy while being digested.
- The foundation of ignorance, doubt, pessimism, ...
- Examples : foods that have been strongly processed, canned or frozen and/or are old, stale or incompatible with each other - meat, fish, eggs and liquor are especially tamasic.

A Yoga sadhaka can survive easily on sattvic foods alone. Householders that live in the world and have to keep pace with its' changes also need rajasic energy. They ought to keep a balance between the sattvic and rajasic foods and try to avoid tamasic foods as much as possible.

5.6 Obstacles and personal development and Yoga

In order to grow and live a healthy life on the Yoga path of
physical, mental, emotional and spiritual development, and obtain
maximum benefit, the practitioner needs to know and become
aware of the obstacles that he is going to come face to face with,
which may disrupt the Yoga and health journey. This will enable
a Sadhaka / practirioner to understand about life challenges or
problems. Remember to transcend body, mind and emotions
one has to know and understand them first. Yoga is being skilful
in action and to be prepared and preventive now, rather then to
repair and repent later on.
In modern times where we are living life full of destructive
stimulants, sensory bombardments, spinal reflex conditioning or
competitive attitude where we face these challenges or obstacles
and get stressed, feel depressed and low mood. In ancient times
in Shiva- Samhita- Three hundred years ago Great unknown Rishi
and author of the Shiva-Samhita cautioning his disciples by the
following verses- "there are many hard and almost insurmountable
obstacles in Yoga, yet the Yogi should go on with his practice at
every obstacle and problem; even were his life to come to the
throat." Its such a beautiful message for all of us modern people
to live our life with not compromising with our values, morals,
health and well being in any situation. Taking every situation as an
opportunity and not as a problem can help us to be more and more
positive, confident and enthusiastic towards our health and well
being.
In Shiva Samhita is also stated that the inner journey to the Self
or Consciousness is not always easy. Its so true in our general life.
There will be many obstacles to face and overcome if you want
to be happy and healthy. There's no denying that Yoga practice
and following the right path in beginning can be frustrating or
disappointing at times. Your situation, society, work, etc might
be not supporting your health and Yoga practice, but you should
always adhere to your health and well being in all and every

situation. Your strong will and commitment with awareness will help you to deal with the obstacles.

In a sense, obstacles are defence mechanisms of body and mind against the process of self development or transcending body, mind and emotional conditioning. They're part of our mental conditioning historically or addiction of living with problems, suffering and miseries holding us away from experiencing the higher self and preventing us from pushing our practice along too quickly to be free and enjoy the higher bliss. These defence mechanisms result in obstacles when one quit away from healthy yogic life; ignore the body, mind and emotions; not understanding nature of mental process and destructions.

Probably the best-known traditional obstacles are the nine listed in the first chapter of the Yoga-Sutra (1.30): The first, sickness (vyadhi), is a physical obstacle. The other eight are mental obstacles- languor (styana), doubt (samshaya), heedlessness (pramada), sloth (alasya), dissipation (avirati), false vision (bhranti-darshana), nonattainment of yogic stages (alabdha-bhumikatva), and instability in these stages (anavasthitatva).

Vyadhi: Disease or Sickness - This first Yoga obstacle refers to physical illnesses. Following your healthy living and practising Yoga when health is not good, for whatever reason, is always more difficult for Sadhaka. One of the reasons behind origin as well as growth of Hatha-Yoga as a system itself was to gain health, fitness, and vitality so Sadhakas or followers were being able to prevent or cure all the physical, mental and emotional diseases. Following a well balanced and healthy life style, vegetarian nutritional diet, balance of rest and exercise, positive thinking, contemplations and visualisation as part of Yoga practices, will ensure the Vyadhi obstacle is overcome.

Styana: Languor- The next significant obstacle on the Yoga journey is an advanced state of apathy. This apathy diminishes your willingness to practice Yoga and commit to your responsibilities. It can lead to neglect and reluctance to practise Yoga in the way it should to be practised to get much out of it. In general life here we tend to ignore and neglect all our responsibilities, no interest in work or even general things we need to do.

Sanshaya: Doubt - Next obstacle is doubting the benefits and stages of Yoga practices. This comes when you have low self esteem. There are two kinds of doubt. In the first kind the one may doubt the practice or resources. This can be due to having people around being judgmental and leaving negative impressions about you. Not allowing you to be judged through others perception can help overcome it. The second kind of doubt is self-doubt. Here the one looses faith in his/her own self. Positive thinking, finding your own skills and strengths, keep following your healthy path and self-belief can help to overcome this obastacle.

Pramada: Heedlessness- The 4th Yoga obstacle, Pramada, occurs when the Sadhaka lacks care and negligence takes over the health well being and Yoga Sadhana. Health and well being is combination physical, mental, emotional, spiritual as well as social and economical responsibilities skilfully requires a unique approach and attitude. If Sadhaka doesn't have the proper emotional and mental attitudes, it might turn the positive aspects of a personality into negative ones.

Alasya: Sloth- One cannot attain goal in life with lazy and inert state of mind and body. It is hard to deal with ones own will power, and this arouses Alasya or laziness. The path to Yoga or healthy life success is tough most of the time in beginning, and strong will power can support you along the way. As our master Swamij Gitanada Giri states that Yoga path is like 'walking the razors edge'. A passive approach will almost certainly lead to a slow and ineffective advance so the Sadhaka should approach an active and conscious healthy yogic approach to avoid or overcome this obstacle.

Avirati: Dissipation- next obstacle is indulgence in the material world and pleasures. Physical objects hold a magnetic attraction to almost every one. Yoga demands you to let go of these material desires and be free of worldly attachments to progress in the realm of the spiritual evolution. In context of healthy living one gets indulged or addicted to problems and health issues for sympathy or attention. Many people will say my stress, my depression, my asthma, my obesity, and these problems becomes their possessions. Learn to let go and as Swamiji sated that "health and happiness are your birthrights."

Bhrantidarshan: False vision- When ever we get stuck in our negativity, ideas, concepts and actions we found ourselves failed, we tend to be in this state we perceive ourselves as a week, negative, low mood and unsuccessful person, on other hand it can be over-confidence and denying our realities as that also results in frustration. Try to look positively and observe various situations without being judgmental and conditioned by yourselves or other people. Also keeping your hopes and expectations in close contact with reality will be a great help.

Alabdha-bhumikatva- This Yoga obstacle, Alabdha-bhumikatva, often arises when a Sadhaka is not achieving the desired goals on the Yoga path. It takes a long time to come out of the shell of mental conditioning and experience higher stages as well as also being victims of our own discouragement. When a failure occurs we fall into a state of self-deprecation, accompanied by pessimism. Failing to reach a step on your path to achieve your ideals can lead to worst forms of this Yoga obstacle. To overcome this obstacle Sadhaka has to keep repeating his Yoga and health practices, regularly in rhythm. Our Master Amma always says "do your best and leave the rest".

Anavasthitatva: Instability- Many times we get to hear from our students in first session that, "I've never done anything as incredible as this before." "Yoga is changing my whole life." You are a great teacher and I am so pleased to find you in the end". After this promising start, the Sadhaka slips back to what he considers to be a lower level of practice or miseries of life. Patanjali named obstacle as 'anavasthitva'- instability or unsteadiness. We all start new things with big promises and hopes beyond our reality and capabilities. Understanding our limitations, capabilities, skills and availability of time and being responsible and kind can help overcome and avoid this obstacle in our life.

Yoga-Sutra 1.31. Duhkha-daurmanasya-angam-ejayatva-shvasa-prashvasah vikshepa-sahabhuva. Patanjali states that these obstacles result in four distractions (vikshepa): suffering or distress (duhkha), depression or melancholy (daurmanasya), physical restlessness (angam-ejatva), and disturbed breathing (prashvasah). These distractions are signs that something is wrong or imbalanced with your practice.

These four distractions arise as a consequence of the nine obstacles described in the previous sutra. If you try to look into your own life then these distractions are easy to notice. When you find yourself under influence one of these, you need to find out what's going on in subtler levels and work it out. Sadhaka can notice how easy it is to observe when someone is experiencing pain, dejection, restlessness of body, or irregularities of breath (the four of this sutra). You may not be able to know the root cause, but you can sure spot the symptom on the surface.

Overcoming obstacles by meditation- Observe our own body gestures, body language, general level of pain and mood, mental and emotional activities and you can easily see if something is going on at the subtler level. Try to find out what is distracting you and how it is disturbing your Yoga practice, health and well being as distraction is followed by disturbance. In Sutra 1.32 Maharishi Patanjali describes the solution to the obstacles, which is 'single pointed concentration, or meditation (dhyana). Sadhaka must choose one of the suitable object's for meditation.

Yoga Sutra 1.32 tat-pratisedha-artham-eka-tattva-abhyasah

For preventing and overcoming obstacles and their resultants Sadhaka should practice or cultivate the habit to focus on single object or principle. As if mind is focused then its less likely to be lost in worldly maya/illusion of destruction resulting into disturbances. There are many tools/ objects or principles to focus, meditate or contemplate to attain the stage of single pointed awareness or meditation. One has to keep following the right path, for holistic health and well being on all level in every moment.

How to Work with Obstacles- In the beginning of your Yoga and health journey even before you come to face these obstacles try to understand yourself, your strengths as well as weakness to avoid these obstacles. Now the first thing to find out is 'Am I ready to start my Yoga journey'? Find out how much time I am going to put in it. Then think about what is involved in following the Yoga path. Many Sadhakas realize that, after a few sessions of half-hearted practice, they don't really feel fit for the Yoga path. They may not be interested in Yoga practices. They may not have the time for Yoga or may be not able to give up worldly pleasures that are not allowed on the serious Yoga path. They might have to spend the time on another responsibility in their lives, or they may not see the point of the Yoga practice. If you find you are not ready then let the practice go and wait for the right time or make an easy and practical space for Yoga in your life and bring the changes gradually with patience. This can also be seen and considered in all the other practices or opportunities and challenges you are taking on.

If you are ready to start, then the next step is to accept yourself as you are with love and respect - even your ignorance. In beginning of the Yoga- Vashishtha it is stated that one who is not too ignorant and one who is not enlightened is eligible to study this scripture, allow yourself to accept that there is much more to learn, practice and realize and you are not all knowing. By accepting mental processes and ignorance you can weaken their power or allow them to be dissolved. This ignorance/ avidya is in respect of consciousness rather then knowledge or intelligence. According to Swamiji ignorance is not only lack or knowledge or understanding but highest level or ignorance is denying the truth. So accept your truth and start working on all the aspects of your personality you are finding need to be changed or improved.

Ramana Maharshi said, "Every living being belongs to be always happy, untainted by sorrow; and everyone has the greatest love for himself, which is solely due to the fact that happiness is his real nature. Hence, in order to realize that inherent and untainted happiness . . . it is essential that he should know himself. For obtaining such knowledge, the enquiry Who am I? In quest of the Self is the best means."

Faith- in the righteousness of what you are doing as well as in your strength or ability to attain the success in your life will keep motivating you in moments of distraction. "The person who has control over himself attains verily success through faith; none other can succeed. Therefore, with faith, Yoga should be practiced with care and perseverance." (Shiva-Samhita). Follow your health, heart and intuitions with faith and self-belief.

Intention- Your clear intention and constant mindfulness (smirti) of what you are doing and why, in regard to both short-term and long-term goals and in the subtle adjustments of everyday practice will help you to prevent as well as prepare to deal with the obstacles.

Contentment (samtosha)- Being realistic and accepting both success and failure with grace, and self-respect; and also willingness to take risks and embrace uncertainty will prevent you from disappointment. "As long as one is not satisfied in the self, he will be subjected to sorrow. With the rise of contentment the purity of one's heart blooms. The contented man who possesses nothing owns the world." **(Yoga-Vashishtha)**

Discrimination (viveka)- Carefully discriminating (viveka) between what's right and wrong or using discernment in your healthy living as to what is important what is not. Avoiding them will keep you safe from obstacles. Swamiji mentioned that if you want to enjoy health and well being then stop avoiding good (virtuous) for pleasure.

Svadhyaya- awareness of body, mind, and emotions can keep you notifying yourself about ongoing or upcoming obstacles as well as their results. "By listening to instructions, by contemplation and by being in the company of a calm and sure-minded preceptor, doubts can be removed." (Shiva-Samhita). Always listen to your body, mind and emotions because if there is any symptoms it simply means you need to pay attention and work on yourself to stay healthy and happy.

Sadhana / practice and Non-attachment or vairajna- Your regular, repetitive and rhythmic practice can lead to success in health, happiness and well being. Swamiji reminds us that if you want to be healthy you have to do healthy things. If you want to be happy do the happy things. This is obvious but so few seem to understand this and complain about their poor health or unhappiness whilst eating junk food or constantly watching depressing TV. Practicing every day to your limits without judging, and holding back is very essential for success. By not being attached to the physical, mental, emotional and material clutter that you don't need, will make your life easier and easier.